THE IgAN COOKBOOK

THRIVING THROUGH FOOD AS AN IGA NEPHROPATHY WARRIOR.

WRITTEN BY

DR. BRUCE A. JULIAN
DR. BLAKE SHUSTERMAN
EMMA RYAN

Disclaimer

This book is intended as a reference only, not as a medical manual. The information provided here is designed to help you make informed decisions about your diet and health. It is not intended as a substitute for the medical advice of physicians or for any treatment that may have been prescribed by your doctor. You should consult a physician regularly in all matters relating to your health. If you suspect that you have a medical condition, you are urged to seek competent medical help. Please consult with your own physician or healthcare specialist regarding suggestions and recommendations made in this book. The use of the book implies your acceptance of this disclaimer.

Mention of specific products, companies, organizations, or authorities in this book does not imply endorsement by the author(s) or publisher, nor does mention of specific products, companies, organizations, or authorities imply that they endorse or are affiliated in any way with this book, author(s), or publisher.

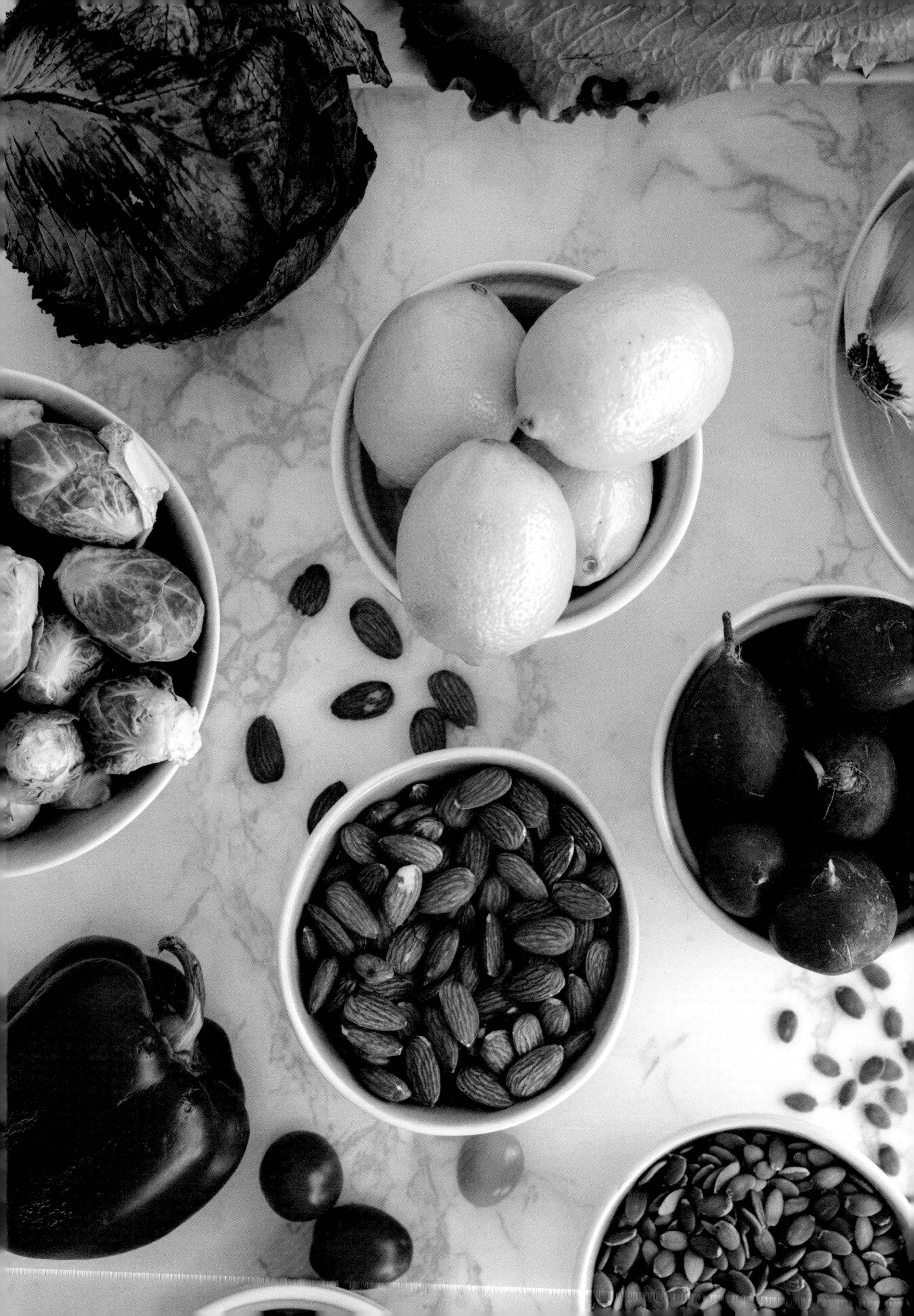

Dr. Bruce A. Julian
Dr. Blake Shusterman
Emma Ryan

First Edition December 2022

Book design by Abby Power
Assisted by Teaspoon Media
Photography by Rachel Maucieri

Notice of Liability: Neither the author(s) nor the IgAN Foundation Inc. shall have any liability to any person or entity for any loss or damage caused or alleged to be caused directly or indirectly by the information contained in this book, or omission from this book.

ISBN: 979-8-9866170-0-8 (Hardcover)
ISBN: 979-8-9866170-1-5 (Softcover)
ISBN: 979-8-9866170-2-2 (e-book)

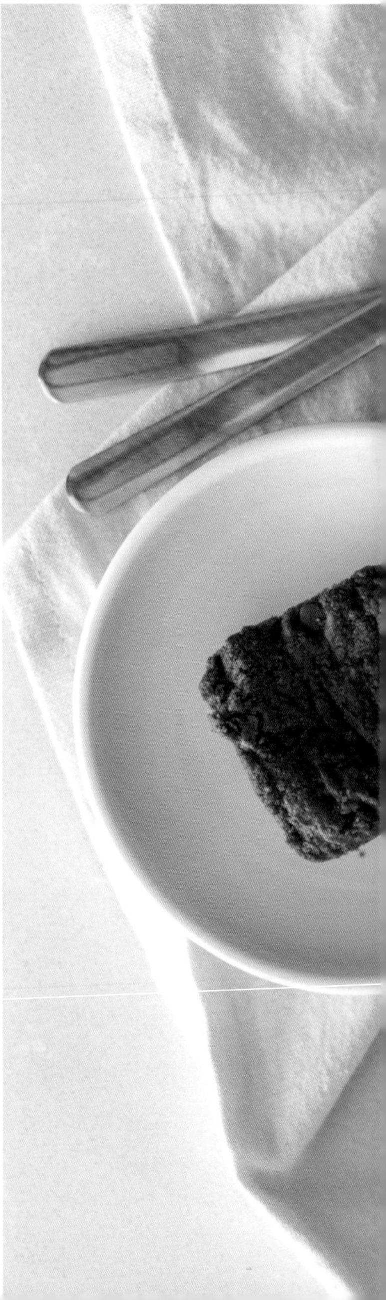

DEDICATED TO:

All the IgA Nephropathy patients and care partners worldwide.

We are kidney WARRIORS!

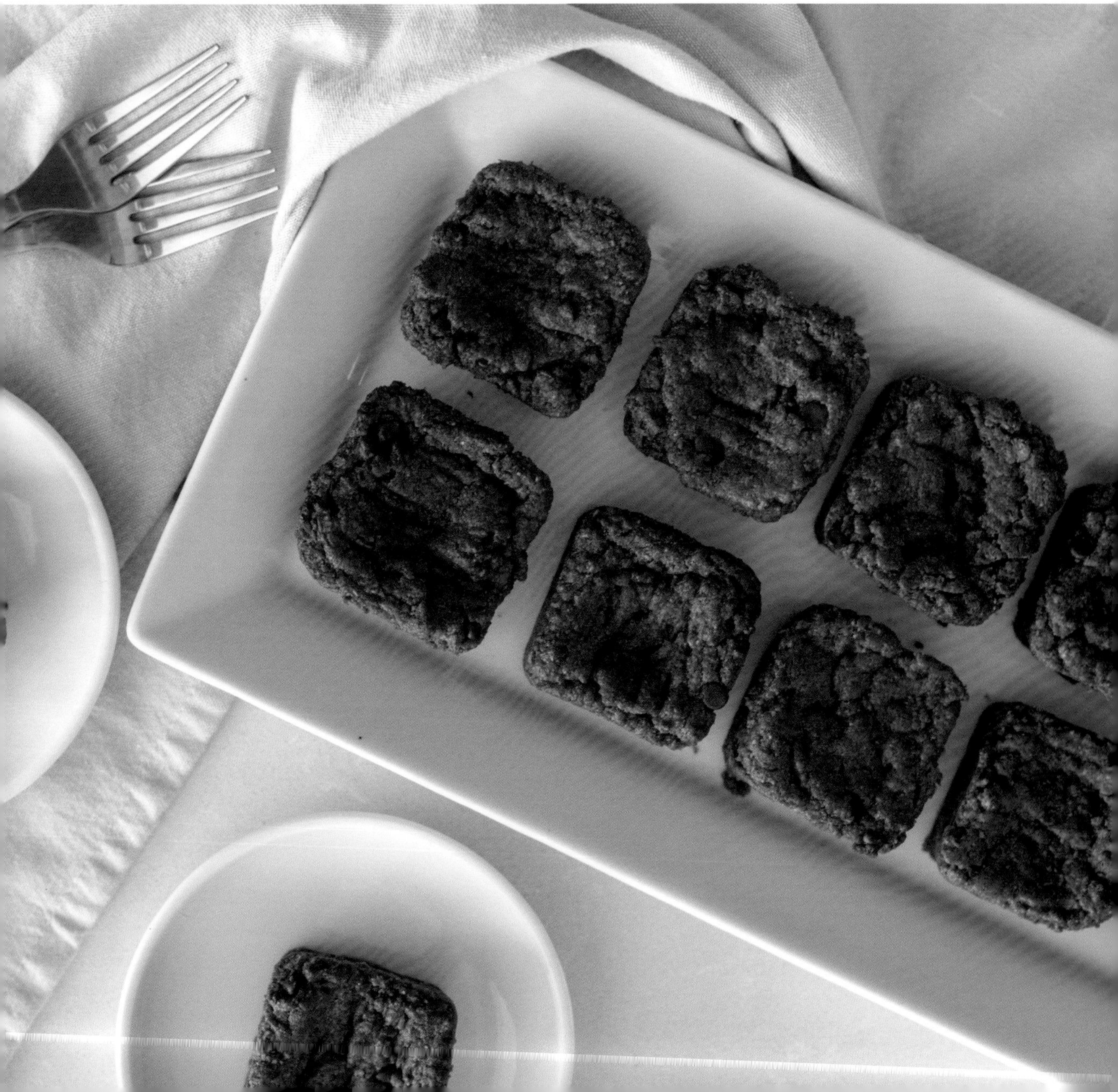

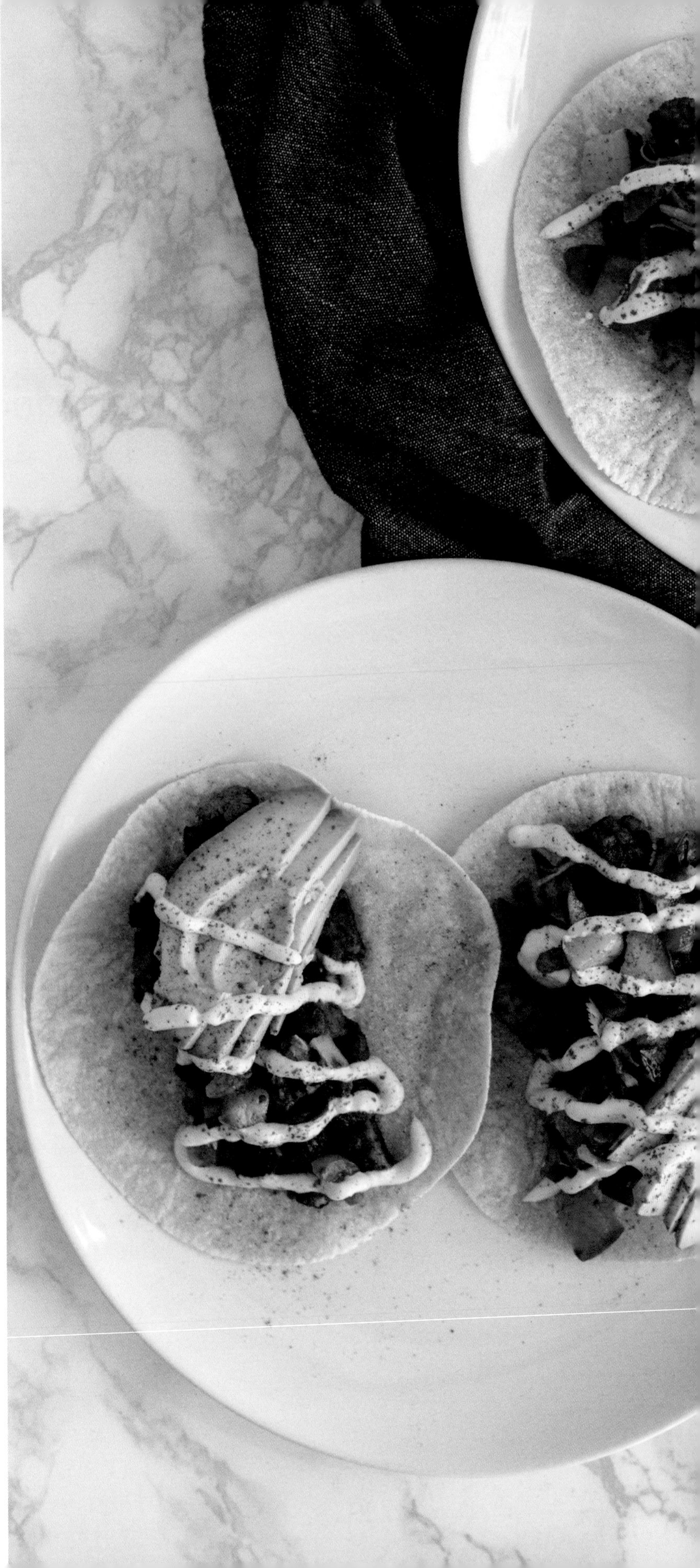

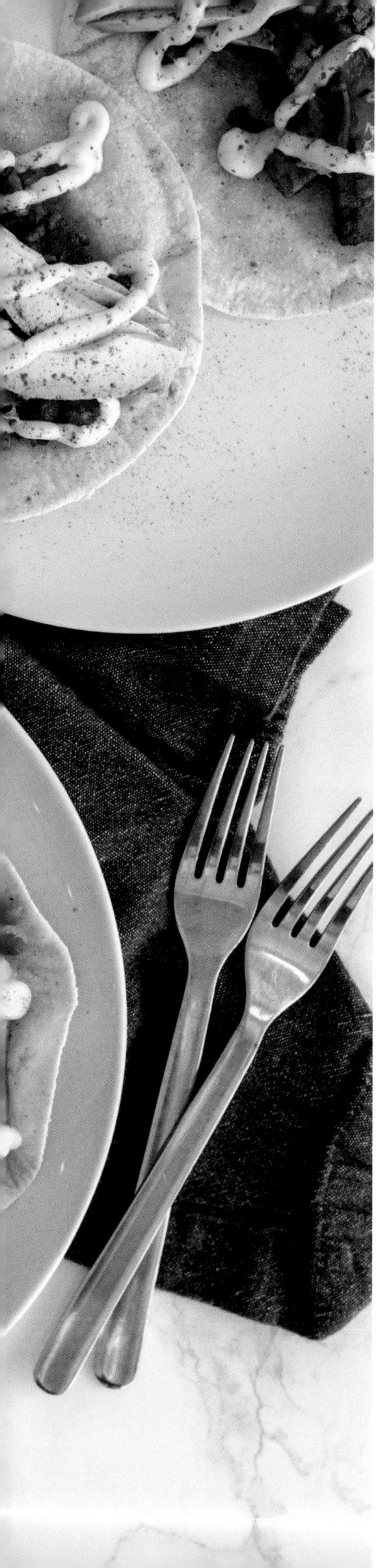

CONTENTS

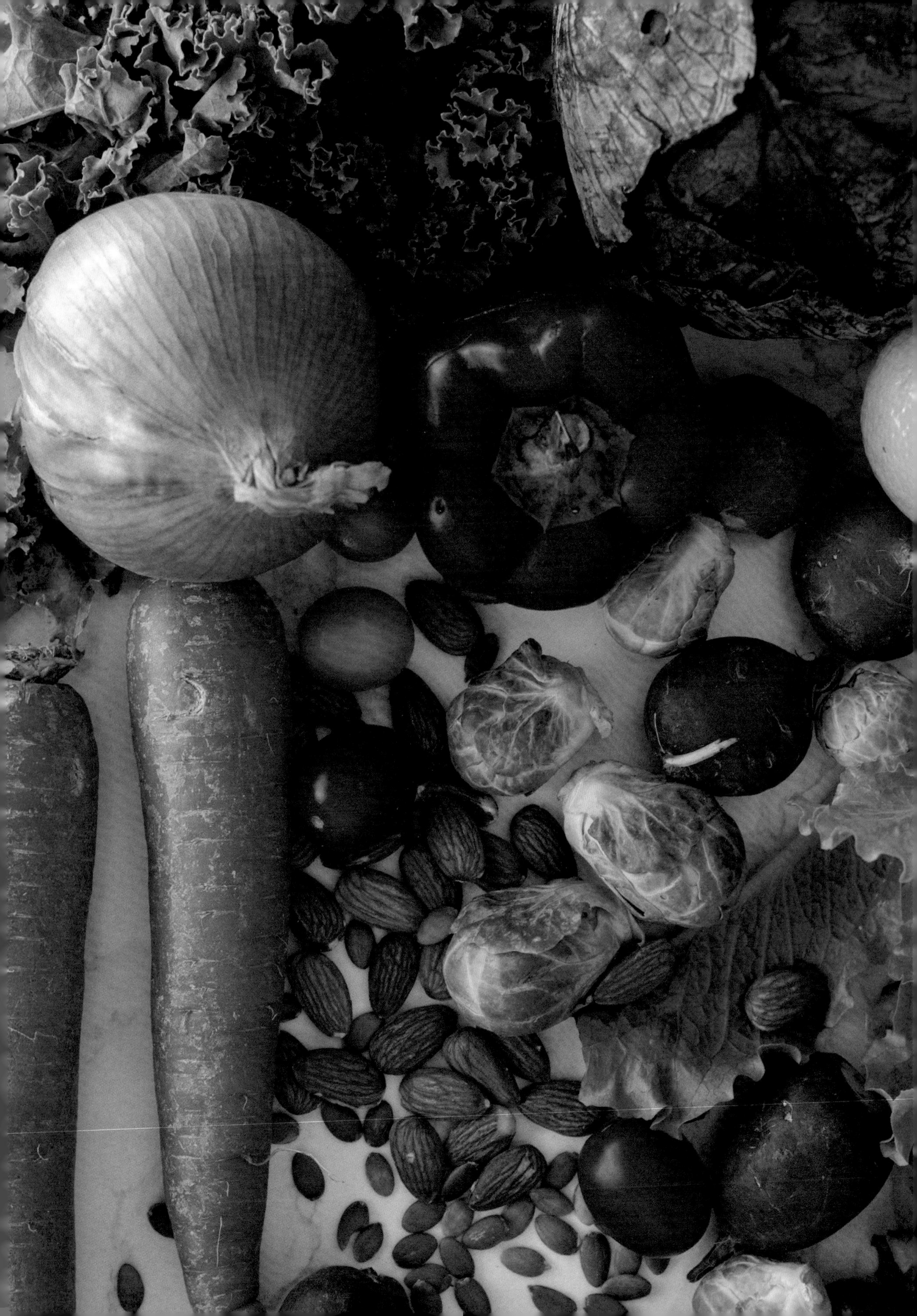

IGA NEPHROPATHY FOUNDATION

MISSION STATEMENT

The IgA Nephropathy Foundation's mission is to be a patient-centric organization focused on finding a cure for IgA Nephropathy. Using the power of the patient community we are focused on funding research, using patient advocacy to empower our patients, and building a network of support.

As a patient run organization, we will work together with the hope of finding better treatment options and the ultimate cure.

By patients, for patients.

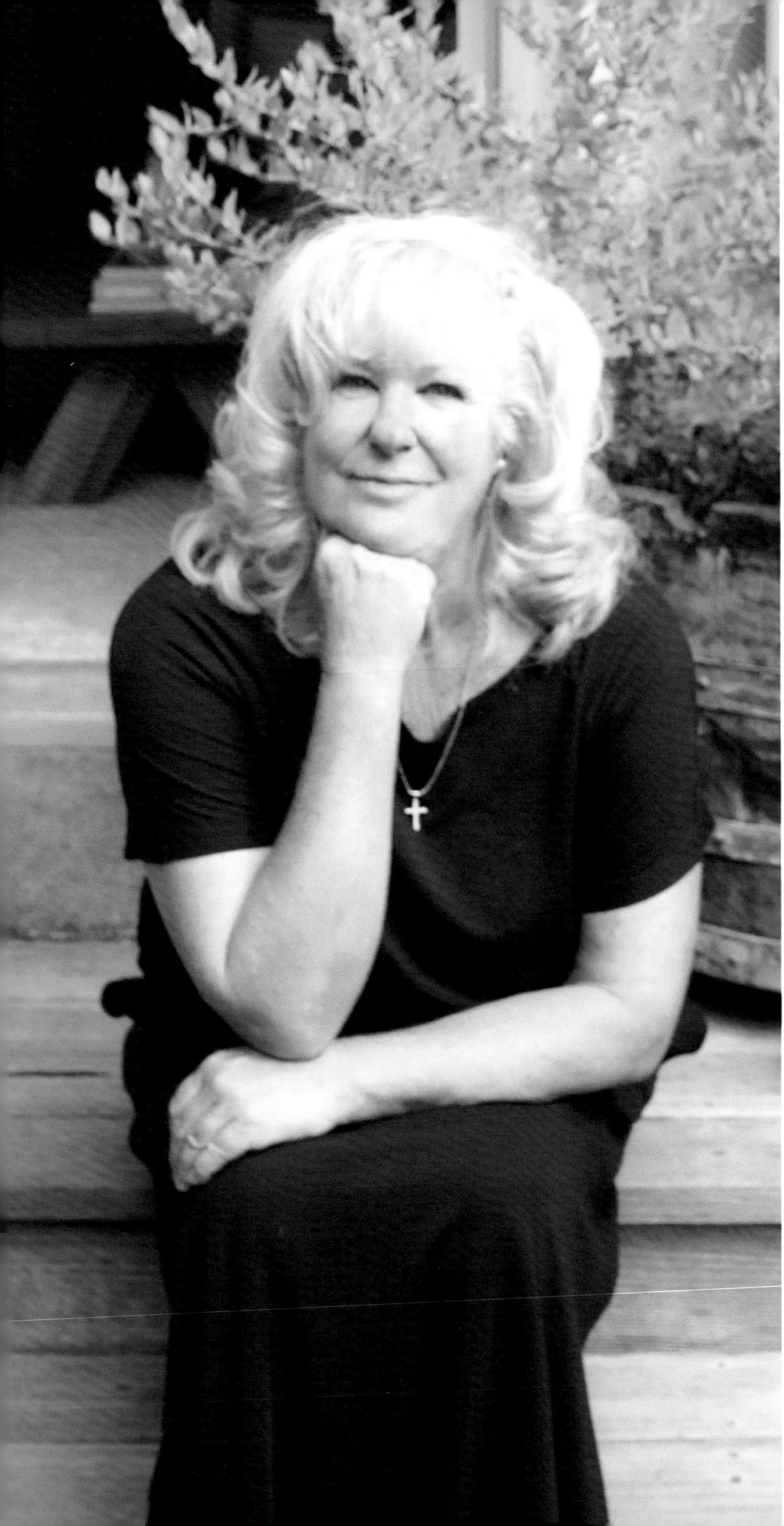

HEY THERE!

I know you likely don't know me, but my name is Bonnie Schneider and I am the founder of the IgA Neprhropathy Foundation. If I met you in person, I'd likely give you a big ole' squeeze as if I was your long-lost best friend, but since we are meeting through this text, I'll have to settle for getting to know you virtually. To start, I want you to know that I am truly honored that you picked up this book and that you're reading along. This book has been a long time in the making for a lot of people and I hope it brings you the peace and inspiration that I was once looking for at the start of my families' IgAN journey. So, before we dive into the nitty and gritty, I'd like to get to know each other. I'll start here, and I hope you'll join me online.

I currently live at the Jersey Shore, where, with my husband Ed, we raised our five amazing children. I'm best known for my home-made jam, my evening cocktails (shh!), walks along the beach, and perhaps talking too much (oops!).

For me, being a mother has always been my greatest joy. Which is why, in 2004, when our 13-year-old son Eddie was diagnosed with IgA Nephropathy, my world turned upside down. Although IgAN is the most common glomerular kidney disease, as most of you reading this might understand, receiving this diagnosis was frightening no matter how "common" they said it was. At the time, there was very little information on IgAN. We were desperate to find others who had the same diagnosis, as we felt like we were searching to find someone who could show us how to navigate this new "normal". I thought for sure there would be some type of patient support or advocacy groups, but at the time, there was nothing.

Slowly, but surely my thoughts began to shift. "If we were having such a hard time finding information on IgAN, and there wasn't a place to go or meet other patients and caregivers, then we needed to create that place ourselves." This was the beginning of the IgA Nephropathy Foundation.

Trust me, it didn't happen overnight, but it became my purpose. I knew we couldn't have been alone, and I so badly wanted to create a community that could foster the support and care that patients, care-givers, and families needed. It's now been nearly 18 years in the making, and each day I wake up with the same drive and motivation as I did when we started.

For myself, the creation of the foundation has been an incredible journey not only to serve our patients and care partners but to become the trusted resource for our IgAN community. We have been built by volunteers and we have grown due to the amount of love this community has poured into it. Most of us understand the struggles because we are all either patients or care partners AND as I like to call it "we have skin in the game."

From our online community, to our annual conference and memberships, it has always been our mission to advocate for and provide education to the IgAN community while also focusing on finding a cure. However, along the way we have heard the cry for more daily support. One of the many hurdles that this community continues to ask about is "What can I eat?" And so here we are, with our very first "IgA Nephropathy Cookbook".

As you read through this book you will hear from trusted medical resources about living with IgAN, patient stories, helpful hints, and you will be introduced to many kidney healthy dishes from around the world. Some of the recipes are from our patients and care partners who have tailored their traditional meals into IgAN friendly options, and some of them will come from my friend, Emma Ryan. Emma is a nutritional health coach and successful owner of two plant-based restaurants, who understands adversity and the need of making good food choices to help us live a longer and healthier life.

So, without further ado, we are excited to share this IgAN cookbook with you! My greatest wish is that something in-between these pages will help you become more mindful about your food, and will give you the resources you need to not only help your battle with kidney disease but also bring you joy in your home-kitchen.

Now, it's your turn to introduce yourself! I would love to hear from you, to hear your story, and to hear how this book is going to be used in your home. Remember, we are always in this together. Come say hello and introduce yourself on our community page at www.facebook.com/IGANFoundation/. I'll be excited to meet you!

And, as always, please feel free to reach out directly at Bonnie@igan.org. I am always here for you.

With love,

Bonnie Schneider

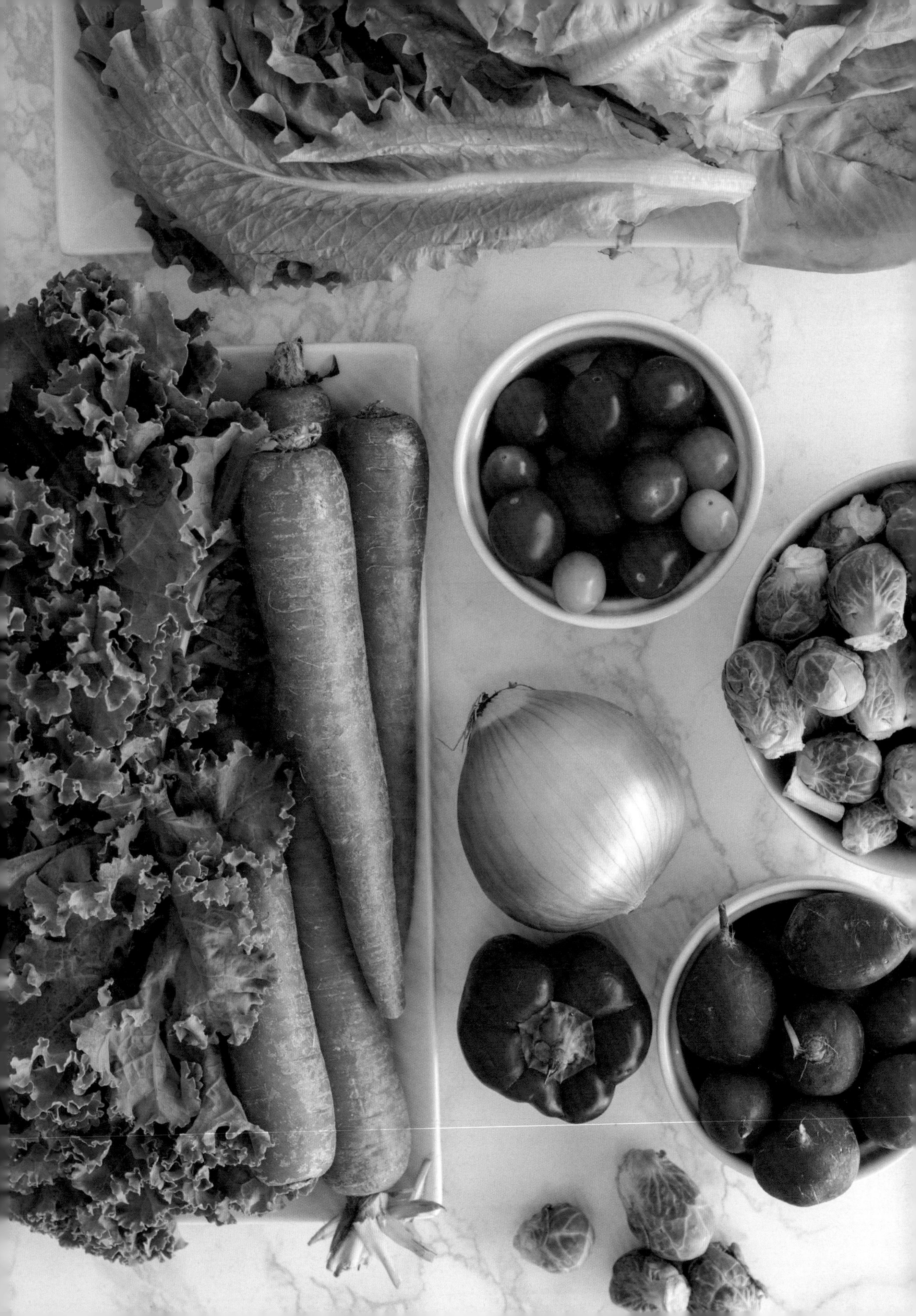

MEET THE AUTHORS

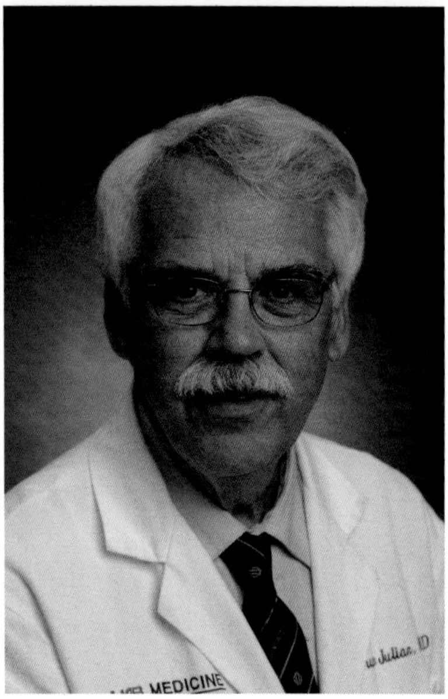

Dr. Bruce A. Julian

Dr. Bruce A. Julian is Professor Emeritus in the Division of Nephrology at the University of Alabama at Birmingham (UAB) who has been treating patients with IgA Nephropathy and investigating the cause of their kidney disease for more than 35 years. His research interest in IgA nephropathy (IgAN) started during his nephrology training at the University of Kentucky where in 1982 he was the first to identify the existence of a hereditary component for some patients with IgAN. This discovery led to his move to UAB in 1984 where he has led and been at the center of much of the scientific progress in the understanding of IgAN as part of the UAB IgAN Research Team. Based on this progress, the UAB IgA Nephropathy Research team in 2011 proposed a multi- step process for the development of IgAN that has become the blue-print for testing new approaches for the treatment of IgAN.

In 1987 Dr. Julian was a founding member of the IgA Nephropathy Club that later became the International IgA Nephropathy Network to organize multiple international symposia for researchers to exchange ideas. He was a member of the international group that developed the Oxford Classification of the pathology features of IgAN. In 2013 Dr. Julian received the UAB Max Cooper Award for Excellence in Research. In 2015 he co-founded Reliant Glycosciences, LLC, a biotechnology company focused on the development of biomarker assays for IgAN. Dr. Julian has published 145 papers and 18 book chapters on IgAN.

Dr. Blake Shusterman

Dr. Blake Shusterman is a board-certified nephrologist and partner at Carolina Nephrology, a twenty-two-provider practice in Greenville, SC. He is also the creator of The Cooking Doc (www.thecookingdoc.co), and author of the book The Cooking Doc's Kidney-Healthy Cooking: A Modern 10-Step Guide to Preventing and Managing Kidney Disease.

Dr. Shusterman serves as the medical director at multiple dialysis units that provide in-center dialysis, home hemodialysis, peritoneal dialysis and acute, in-hospital dialysis. He is a Clinical Assistant Professor at the USC School of Medicine in Greenville and oversees the medical student nephrology rotations.

In the past he has served as president at Carolina Nephrology and currently he is a board member of the Carolina Kidney Alliance. He is passionate about home dialysis, patient education, and the importance of diet in the management of chronic kidney disease. Dr. Shusterman earned his medical degree from The Ohio State University and went on to complete his internal medicine residency and nephrology fellowship at the University of Virginia where he served as chief fellow. He holds a BA in Anthropology from Tufts University.

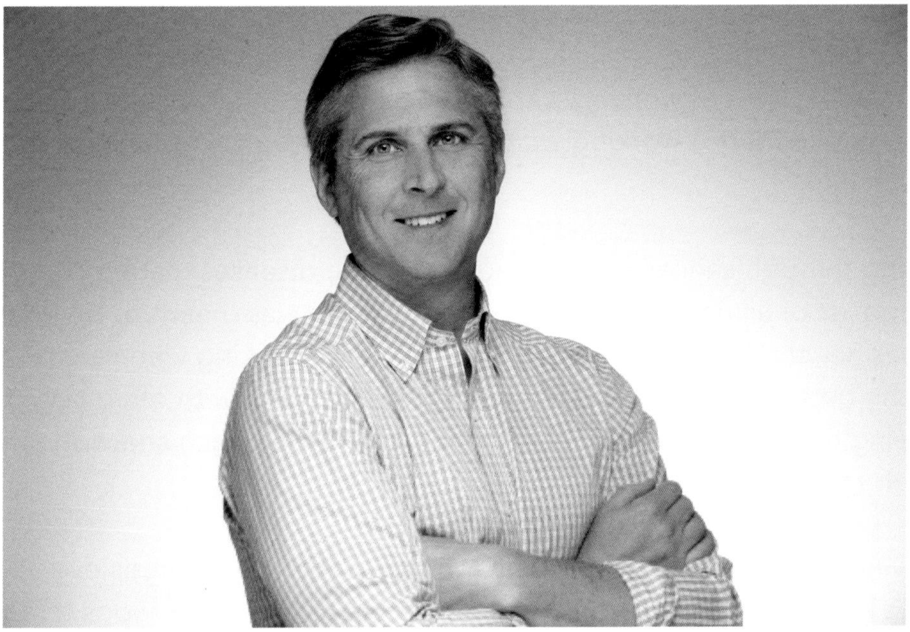

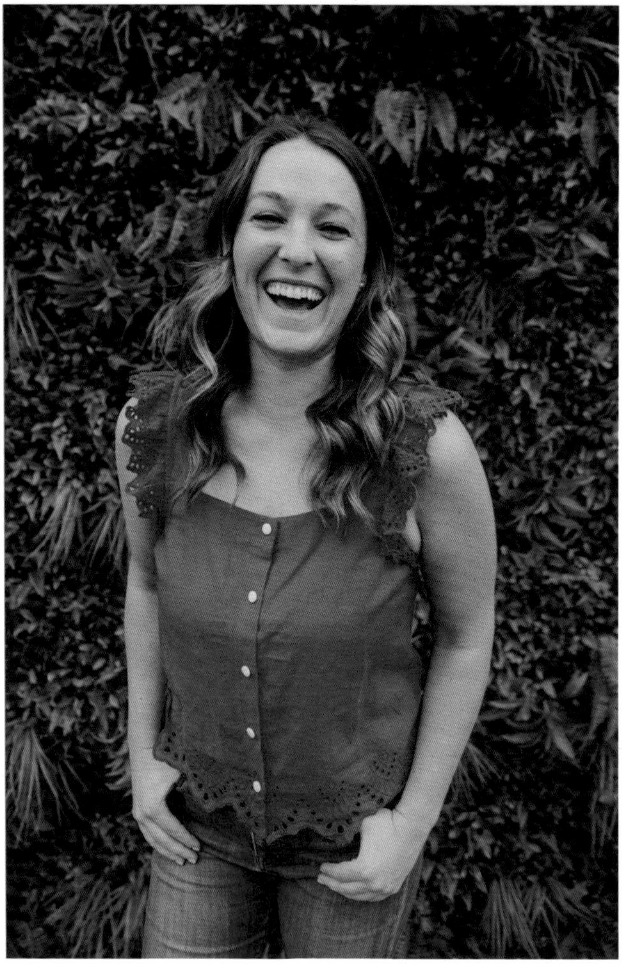

Emma Ryan

Emma Ryan is a plant-based chef, integrative nutrition health coach, and the founder & owner of Plant, a plant-based restaurant concept in Oklahoma. While she specializes in working with people with auto-immune diseases, she has years of experience working with individuals of all backgrounds and dietary needs.

After living through cancer, multiple auto-immune diseases, eating disorders, and a long list of ailments, she realized that this life was meant to be lived, and it was her choice how she was going to live it. Working with clients means she gets to share her love of health and wellness with other people while being their accountability partner and being the coach she wished she had when she needed it most.

She is living proof that changing the way we eat and live changes everything, and she's here to help you find comfort in eating plant-based foods that fuel you for your adventures ahead.

ACKNOWLEDGEMENTS

There are several amazing individuals whose talents and caring made this book possible, we thank you from the bottom of our hearts. This book would not have been possible without you.

Bonnie Schneider for being the inspiration that drove the creation of this cookbook. It was her dream to bring this book to life and her passion that drove the process from beginning to end.

Brian Parlato for his project planning skills and bringing all the elements of the book together.

Lauren Levy for developing the nutrition data for each recipe and all her suggestions to make each recipe as healthy as possible for IgAN patients.

Abby Power for her creativity and talent in designing the look and feel of this beautiful book.

Rachel Maucieri for her gorgeous photographs of each recipe.

THANK YOU

to our wonderful partners in the battle against
IgA Nephropathy whose generous support helped make
this book a reality.

ALNYLAM PHARMACEUTICAL

CALLIDITAS THERAPEUTICS

CHINOOK THERAPEUTICS

NOVARTIS

OMEROS

OTSUKA / VISTERRA

TRAVERE THERAPEUTICS

VERA THERAPEUTICS

Alnylam®
PHARMACEUTICALS

calliditas
THERAPEUTICS

CHINOOK
THERAPEUTICS

NOVARTIS

OMEROS®

Otsuka | Visterra
Otsuka Group of Companies

TRAVERE™
THERAPEUTICS

vera
therapeutics

GLOSSARY

ACEi AND ARB

Angiotensin-converting enzyme inhibitors (ACEi) and angiotensin II receptor blockers (ARB) are medications that are helpful for IgAN patients. They can be used to reduce blood pressure and proteinuria, and slow progression of kidney damage. There are possible complications, especially when used together, so ongoing discussions with your doctor or medical practitioner are important when using them.

ALBUMIN TO CREATININE RATIO

The urine albumin-to-creatinine ratio (ACR) is a measurement of the amount of a specific protein (albumin) leaking from the blood through the kidneys into the urine compared to the amount of creatinine, a waste product excreted by the kidneys, in the same urine specimen. The ACR is used to estimate the amount of albumin excreted in 24 hours. The recommended method of testing is to use a spot urine sample. The higher the ACR level, the more severe the kidney disease. A normal urine ACR is less than 30 milligram albumin per gram creatinine (mg/g); a ratio of 30–300 mg/g is moderately increased (historically known as microalbuminuria) and below the level of detection by tests for total protein; and ACR values above 300 mg/g are severely increased (historically known as macroalbuminuria). An ACR above 300 mg/g for more than three months indicates chronic kidney disease.

ALBUMINURIA

Albuminuria is a sign of kidney disease and means you have too much of the protein albumin in your urine. Albumin is the most abundant protein in the blood. A healthy kidney doesn't let much albumin pass from the blood into the urine.

ANTIBODY

An antibody is a protein that recognizes foreign substances, like bacteria and viruses, and neutralizes them. After exposure to a foreign substance, called an antigen, antibodies continue to circulate in the blood or be in various secretions (such as in the nose), providing protection against illness due to future exposures to that antigen.[1]

CKD

Chronic kidney disease (CKD) means there has been an abnormality of the function or structure of the kidneys for at least three months[5]. There are five stages of CKD based on GFR that are subdivided into three groups based on the amount of albuminuria.

CORTICOSTEROIDS

Corticosteroids are steroid hormones made in the adrenal glands or they can be made synthetically. There are two types: glucocorticoids and mineralocorticoids. Several glucocorticoids can reduce inflammation and are used to treat IgAN in some cases. They also come with various side effects that can limit their use. The most used synthetic glucocorticoid is prednisone. Corticosteroids are not anabolic steroids, which are performance-enhancing drugs used by some athletes and bodybuilders.

CREATININE

Creatinine is a waste product from the normal wear and tear of muscles in your body and from some foods. Your kidneys remove creatinine from your blood. Doctors measure the amount of creatinine in your blood to estimate your GFR. As kidney disease gets worse, the level of creatinine goes up.[3]

CYSTATIN C

Cystatin C is a protein that is produced by the cells in your body. When the kidneys are working well, they keep the level of cystatin C in your blood low. A high level of cystatin C in your blood may mean that your kidneys are not working well. The serum cystatin C level can be used with or without the level of creatinine in the same serum sample for calculation of eGFR.

DIALYSIS

Dialysis is a treatment procedure that filters waste products and removes water from your blood, as your kidneys did when they were healthy. There are two main types of dialysis: hemodialysis and peritoneal dialysis.

ELECTROLYTE

An electrolyte is a substance that breaks up into particles with electrical charges when it is dissolved in water or body fluids. Some electrolytes are important minerals—like sodium, calcium, phosphorus, and potassium—that are critical to many functions in the body. Electrolyte irregularities are common with kidney diseases because the kidneys play a key role in maintaining normal blood levels of most electrolytes. Malfunctioning kidneys can create high or low blood levels of electrolytes.

FILTRATION

Filtration is the process by which some of the liquid portion of your circulating blood passes through the glomeruli (microscopic filters) in the kidneys to clean the blood. The kidneys filter out certain substances in the blood that the body does not need.[4]

GALACTOSE

Galactose is one of the simple sugars. Sugars can be attached to proteins to make glycoproteins (IgA1 is a glycoprotein that contains galactose).

GLUCOSE

Glucose is one of the simple sugars. It is an important source of energy for your body and is measured by routine blood tests, fingerstick, or a continuous glucose monitoring device. Glucose is often simply called "sugar" in discussions with physicians or health care providers.

GFR, eGFR

Glomerular filtration rate (GFR) is a test that checks how well your kidneys are working. Your kidneys each have about 1,000,000 tiny filters called glomeruli. These filters help remove waste and excess fluid from the blood. A GFR test estimates how much of the fluid portion of your blood passes through these filters each minute. GFR can be measured directly, but requires a complicated test by specialized providers. A mathematical formula that includes your serum creatinine level, serum cystatin C level, or both, as well as your age, weight, height, and sex can be used to calculate the estimated GFR (eGFR). A web-based calculator is available at https://www.kidney.org/professionals/kdoqi/gfr_calculator. Normal eGFR varies according to age, sex, and body size, and declines with age. The measurement is often reported as mL/minute per 1.73 square meters body surface area. The eGFR is a simple test that can provide very accurate results.[2]

GLOMERULAR DISEASE

Glomerular diseases are kidney diseases that damage the glomeruli, often letting protein, red blood cells, or both leak from your circulating blood into the urine. Sometimes a glomerular disease also interferes with the clearance of waste products by the kidney, so they begin to build up in the blood. IgAN is a glomerular disease. Some other common glomerular diseases are focal segmental glomerulosclerosis (FSGS), membranous nephropathy (MN), minimal change disease (MCD), and thin basement membrane nephropathy (TBMN).

GLOMERULUS

Each of your kidneys is made up of about 1,000,000 structural units called nephrons. Each nephron includes a filter, called the glomerulus, which is a specially modified tuft of tiny blood vessels that filters blood in the kidney to create urine. When glomeruli are damaged and can't function as they should, it's called glomerular disease.

HEMATOCRIT

Hematocrit is the percentage of blood volume that is compromised by red blood cells.

HEMOGLOBIN

Hemoglobin is the protein in red blood cells that carries oxygen in the blood.

HEMATURIA

Hematuria is the presence of blood in a person's urine. The two types of hematuria are: macroscopic hematuria (sometimes also termed visible or gross hematuria) when a person can see the blood in the urine and microscopic hematuria when a person needs a microscope to see the blood in urine.3 The measurement for microscopic hematuria is reported as the number of red blood cells (RBCs) seen in a high-power-field view (HPF).[3]

HORMONES

Hormones are substances produced in the body that are transported in tissue fluids such as blood to stimulate specific cells or tissues into action. Several important hormones are produced and regulated by the kidneys. Some of these hormones help control blood pressure, which is why patients are sometimes sent to kidney doctors to help manage their blood pressure. The kidneys produce a hormone called erythropoietin that signals the bone marrow to produce red blood cells. If your kidneys are damaged, you may develop anemia (low hematocrit; low hemoglobin level) if your levels of erythropoietin drop too low.[4]

IMMUNOGLOBULIN

Immunoglobulins are proteins that are also known as antibodies. There are five different types of immunoglobulins: IgG, IgM, IgA, IgD, and IgE.

IGAN

IgAN is the abbreviation for **I**mmuno**g**lobulin **A** **N**ephropathy

INTERNATIONAL IgA NEPHROPATHY PREDICTION TOOLS

For patients with IgAN, a formula can be used to predict at the time of the kidney biopsy the risk of substantial loss of kidney function over intervals up to 80 months. The necessary information includes readily available clinical, laboratory, and kidney-biopsy results at the time of the diagnostic biopsy.
The calculator for adult patients (age 18 years or older at biopsy) is available at https://qxmd.com/calculate/calculator_499/international-igan-prediction-tool-at-biopsy-adults.
The calculator for children is available at https://qxmd.com/calculate/calculator_713/international-igan-prediction-tool-at-biopsy-pediatrics.

KIDNEYS

The kidneys are two bean-shaped organs, each about the size of a fist. They are located near the bottom of the rib cage in the back, one on each side of your spine. Each healthy kidney filters about a half-cup of blood every minute, removing wastes and extra water to make urine. The urine flows from the kidney into a tubular structure called the ureter to drain into the bladder. In removing wastes and extra fluid from your body, your kidneys maintain a healthy balance of water, salts, and minerals—such as sodium, calcium, phosphorus, and potassium—in your blood. They also make hormones that help control your blood pressure, make red blood cells, and keep your bones strong and healthy.[3]

NEPHROLOGIST

A nephrologist is a doctor who diagnoses, treats, and manages patients with acute and chronic diseases that affect the kidney.

NEPHRON

Each of your kidneys is made up of about 1,000,000 filtering structure called nephrons. Each nephron includes a filter, called the glomerulus, and a tubule. The nephrons work through a two-step process: the glomerulus filters your blood, and the cells lining the inside of the tubule reclaim needed substances such as salts, minerals, glucose (sugar), and water that are returned to your blood.[3]

PHOSPHORUS

Phosphorus is a mineral found in many foods, such as beans, nuts, milk, meat, and dark colas. It is also used as a preservative in many processed foods. Damaged kidneys cannot remove phosphorus very well. Too much phosphorus in your blood increases production of a hormone in the parathyroid glands in your neck and of a protein called fibroblast growth factor 23 (FGF23) that can cause problems with the health of your bones and hardening of your arterial blood vessels.

POTASSIUM
Potassium is a mineral and electrolyte found in the body and in many foods. Damaged kidneys cannot remove potassium very well. Too much potassium in your blood is called hyperkalemia and can be dangerous if the level is quite high.

PROTEIN-TO-CREATININE RATIO
The urine protein-to-creatinine ratio is a measurement of how much protein compared to creatinine is in the urine and is measured in a fashion similar to that for the albumin-to-creatinine ratio. It is reported as milligram or gram of protein per gram of creatinine (mg/g or g/g). It is often measured in a spot urine specimen and can be used to estimate the 24-hour total protein excretion. A normal urine protein-to-creatinine ratio is less than 0.5 g/g in children 6 months to 2 years of age, less than 0.25 g/g in children 2-17 years of age, and less than 0.2 g/g in adults (age 18 years and older).

PROTEINURIA
Proteinuria is a sign of kidney disease and means you have too much of protein in your urine. A healthy kidney doesn't let very much protein pass from the blood into the urine. A normal amount of protein in a 24-hour collection of urine is less than 150 mg.

RENAL
Relating to the kidneys.

SERUM
Serum is the liquid in the blood-collection tube after blood has clotted. Serum is used for many routine tests, including measurements of creatinine, electrolytes, and glucose.

TUBULE
Each of the 1,000,000 nephrons in a kidney includes a glomerulus and a tubule. A blood vessel runs alongside the tubule. As the filtered fluid moves

through the tubule, the cells lining the inside of the walls of the tubule reclaim almost all the water, along with minerals and nutrients (including glucose) that your body needs. These cells lining the tubule also deliver excess acid from the body into the fluid in the tubule. The remaining fluid and wastes in the tubule become urine.[3]

TUBULE

Each of the 1,000,000 nephrons in a kidney includes a glomerulus and a tubule. A blood vessel runs alongside the tubule. As the filtered fluid moves through the tubule, the cells lining the inside of the walls of the tubule reclaim almost all the water, along with minerals and nutrients (including glucose) that your body needs. These cells lining the tubule also deliver excess acid from the body into the fluid in the tubule. The remaining fluid and wastes in the tubule become urine.[3]

UROLOGIST

A urologist is a surgical doctor who specializes in the care of patients with disorders of the urinary system.

Disclaimer: All terms and definitions are for reference only and may be incomplete and not tell the whole story regarding your specific medical condition - all medical decisions should be discussed with your doctor or medical practitioner.

1 - Courtesy: National Human Genome Research Institute 2 - Courtesy of MedlinePlus from the National Library of Medicine 3 - National Institute of Diabetes and Digestive and Kidney Diseases (NIDDK) 4 - Courtesy of The Cooking Docs Kidney Healthy Cooking 5- Courtesy of KDIGO

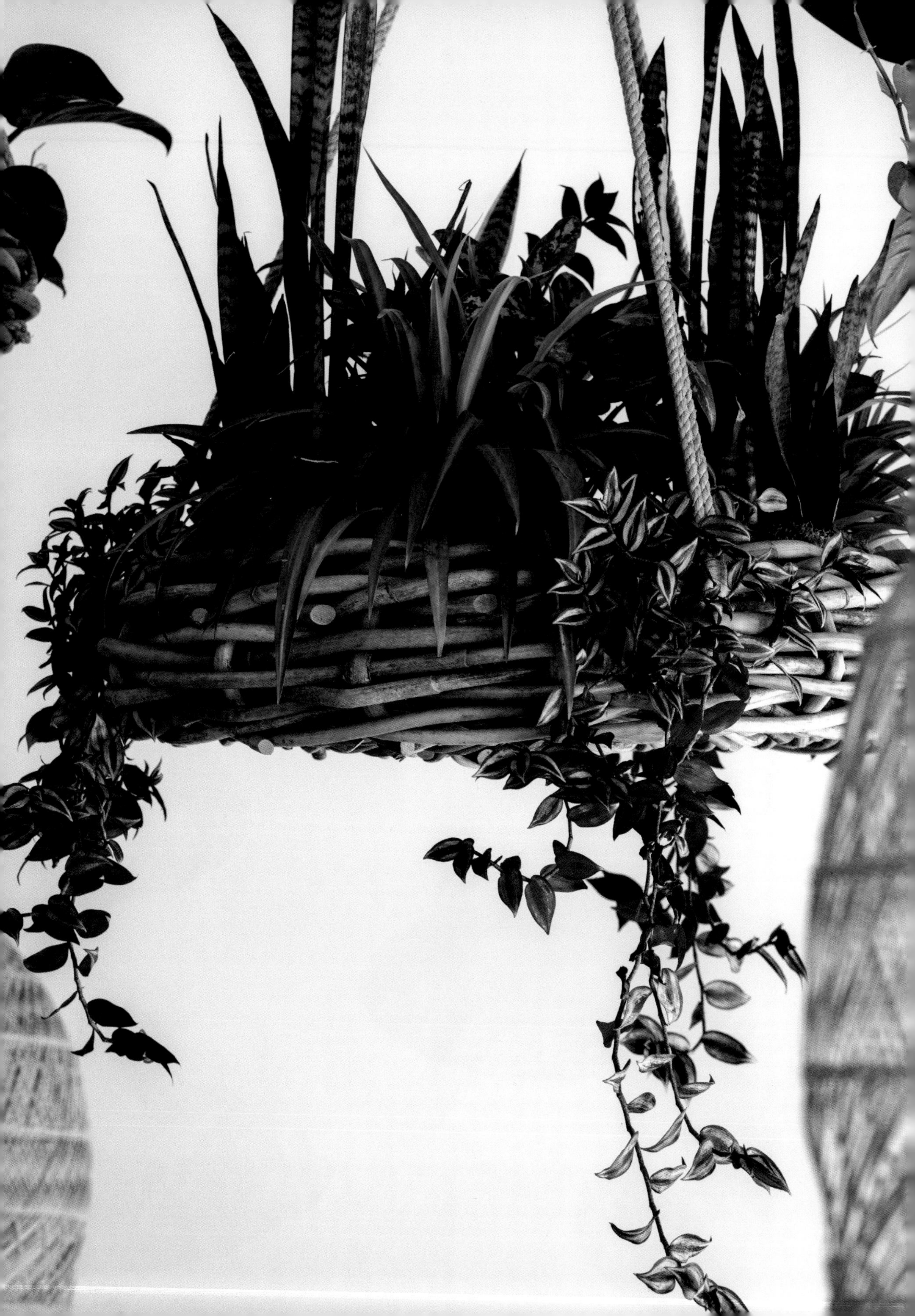

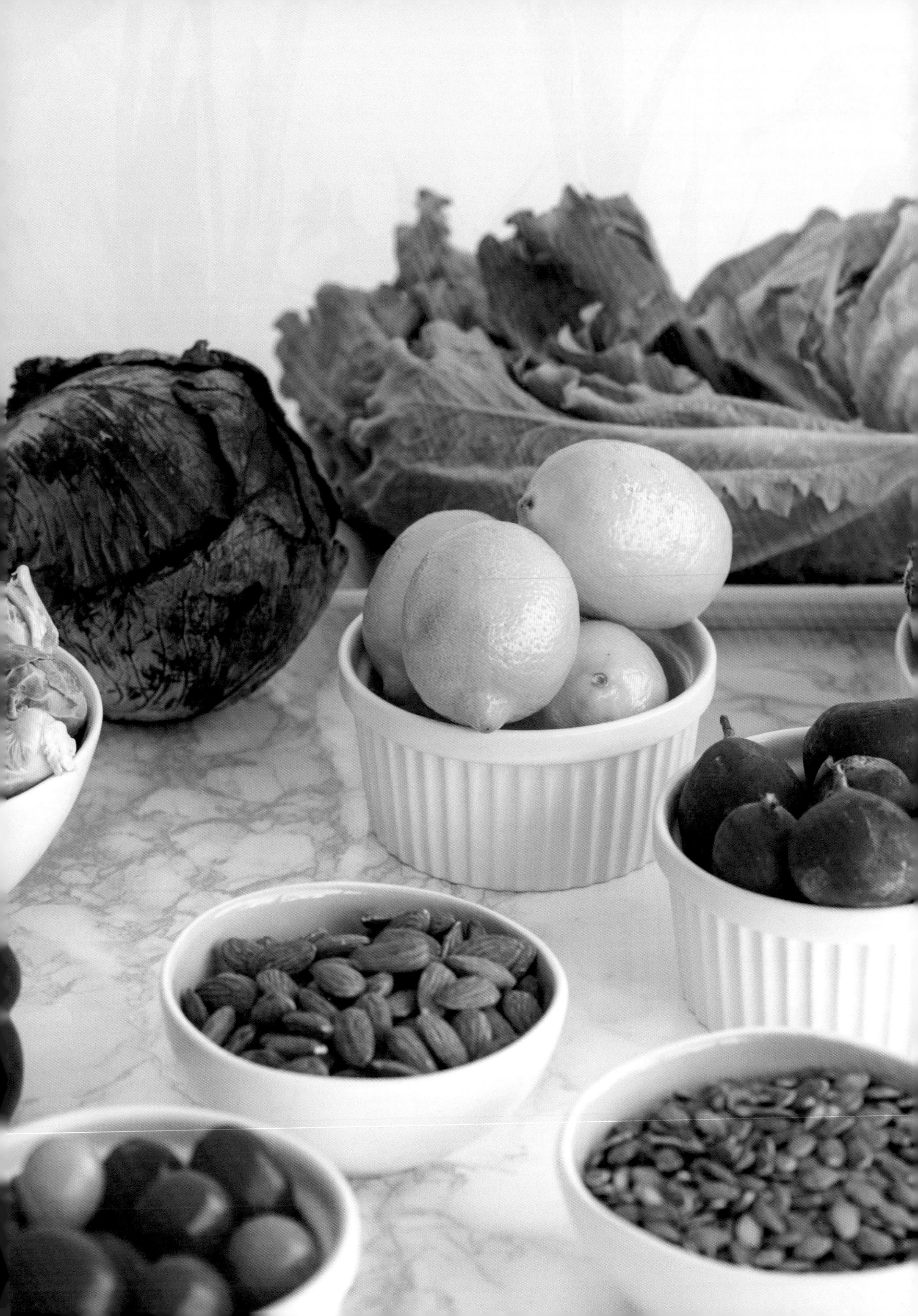

WHAT IS IgAN?

By Dr. Bruce A. Julian

DISCOVERY OF IgA NEPHROPATHY

Immunoglobulin A Nephropathy (IgAN) was first described by French pathologist Dr. Jean Berger and his colleague, Dr. Nicole Hinglais, in 1968 in Paris. New procedures to examine kidney tissue had recently become available to determine whether antibodies in the blood could accumulate in the kidneys to cause damage. These antibodies, also known as immunoglobulins, are proteins made by our immune system to protect us from bacteria, viruses, and other harmful substances in the environment. The immunoglobulins come in different varieties, designated as immunoglobulin A (IgA), immunoglobulin G (IgG), immunoglobulin M (IgM), etc. Drs. Berger and Hinglais were the first to test specifically for the presence of IgA in kidneys.

They examined the kidney tissues of several young adults who had blood in their urine. They were surprised to find IgA had accumulated in large amounts inside their kidneys. Specifically, the IgA was deposited in parts of the kidney called glomeruli—tufts of very small blood vessels that function as the filtering units inside each kidney (Figures 1 and 2). This accumulation of IgA leads to inflammation, and this inflammation damages the structure of these microscopic filters. This damage frequently leads to malfunctioning glomeruli and causes blood and protein to leak into the urine. These conditions are called hematuria (blood in the urine) and proteinuria (protein in the urine). Sometimes the inflammation even leads to a decrease in the kidneys' ability to filter the blood. Poor kidney filtration causes the accumulation of waste products in the blood, such as creatinine (a waste product of muscles and an important test marker for determining kidney health). Doctors use the blood creatinine level to estimate the glomerular filtration rate (eGFR). Reduced kidney filtration can also lead to challenges in maintaining a normal balance of various electrolytes and minerals, including sodium, potassium, calcium, and phosphorus, as well as maintaining the correct water balance in the body.

Kidney Structure

On average, about 1,000,000 nephrons per kidney

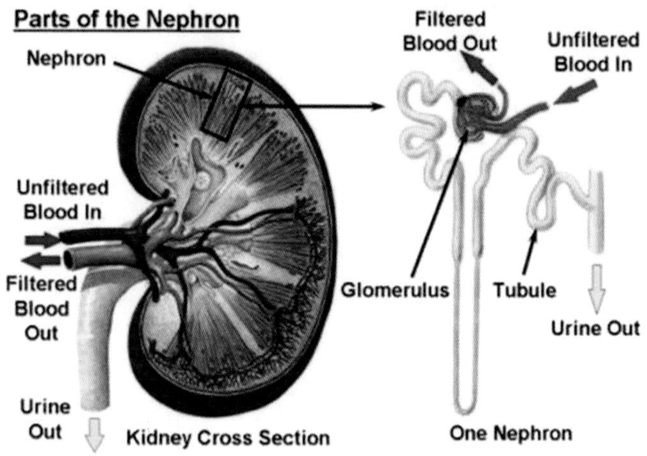

Figure 1.

Structure of the kidney. Unfiltered blood enters the kidney through an artery (top red arrow, left). In the kidney, the artery divides into many smaller vessels to deliver blood to about 1,000,000 nephrons, the functional units of the kidney. Unfiltered blood enters a tuft of tiny blood vessels (capillaries of the glomerulus) where the liquid part of blood is filtered to form urine that flows through a tubule. In the tubule, most of the filtered salt, sugar (glucose), and water are reclaimed to return to the circulating blood. The concentrated urine with waste products then collects in the ureter to leave the kidney (yellow arrow, left).

Normal Glomerulus

Structural Components on Light Microscopy

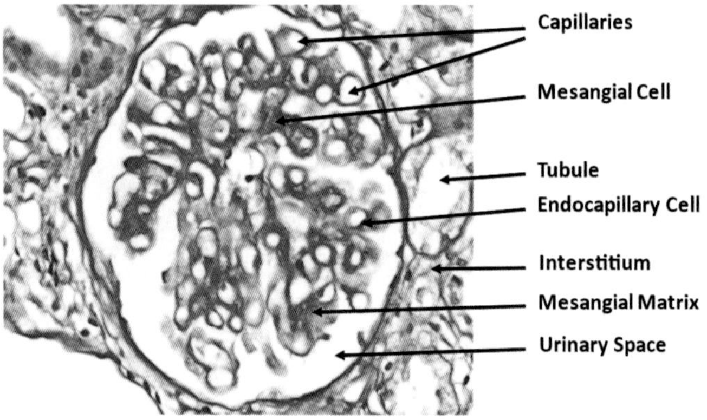

Figure 2.

A thinly cut section of a normal glomerulus after special staining, examined with a microscope at 40-fold magnification. Unfiltered blood circulates through the capillaries (two shown by arrows) in the glomerulus. The fluid portion of the blood filters through the walls of the capillaries to enter the urinary space. The capillaries contain cells (endocapillary cells) and are supported by a framework (mesangial matrix with mesangial cells). The fluid in the urinary space drains through a tubule (connection with the urinary space not shown in this figure) that loops around the glomerulus. The tissue that supports the many tubules is the interstitium.

DIAGNOSIS OF IGA NEPHROPATHY

Even now, more than 50 years since its discovery, IgA Nephropathy still requires a procedure called a kidney biopsy in order to make the diagnosis. This means that there isn't a blood test, urine test, or imaging test (such as a CT scan or ultrasound) that can diagnose IgAN. Instead, a radiologist or nephrologist will have to obtain a tiny sample of the kidney by inserting a needle into one kidney and sending the tissue to a pathologist to examine it. If an abnormal accumulation of IgA (specifically IgA1) is seen in the glomerU-LI (Figure 3), a diagnosis of IgAN is made. Of note, the accumulated IgA1 found in the glomeruli of people with IgAN has a different structure than normal IgA1. This abnormal IgA1 is at the heart of what causes IgA Nephropathy. We will discuss this in greater detail below.

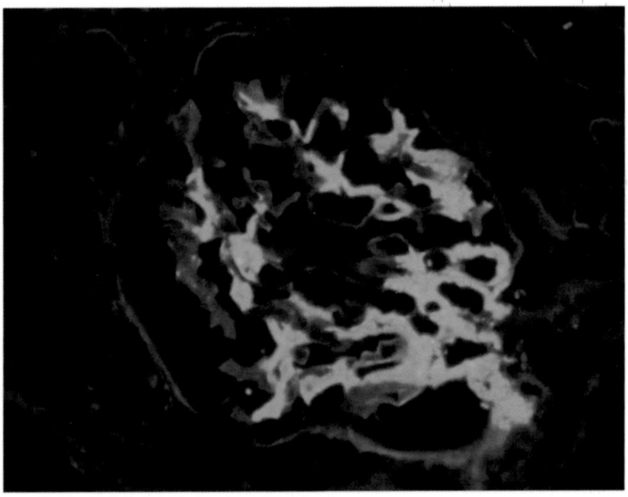

Figure 3.

A thinly cut section of glomerulus of patient with IgAN, stained for IgA and examined with a microscope at 40-fold magnification. The bright green areas indicate IgA that has accumulated in the mesangium.

EPIDEMIOLOGY OF IGA NEPHROPATHY

The frequency of IgAN varies markedly by geographic region. The incidence of newly diagnosed patients per year is about 1 per year per 100,000 persons in the United States but is about 2.5 times higher in Europe and 10 times higher in East Asia. IgA Nephropathy is the diagnosis for about 40-50% of all native-kidney biopsies in Japan, 20-25% in Europe, 10-12% in the United States, and less than 5% in central Africa. Some of this variation is due to differences in health-screening practices and reasons for performing a kidney biopsy; however, genetic factors likely also contribute. In the United States and Europe, the male/female ratio for newly diagnosed patients is about 2.5:1 but about 1:1 in East Asia. The presence of IgA Nephropathy often escapes detection because kidney disease sometimes does not show up in routine laboratory testing. An autopsy study of persons dying from trauma in Finland showed high levels of IgA in the kidneys of 1.3% of the victims. In a study in Japan, 16% of kidney donors, deceased and living, had high levels of IgA in the glomeruli of the donated kidneys at the time of transplantation into the recipient. All donors had shown no evidence of kidney disease during extensive testing prior to surgery. Therefore, the prevalence of IgA Nephropathy may be substantially higher than currently recognized, due to many affected persons having no detected findings of kidney disease.

CLINICAL PRESENTATIONS OF IGA NEPHROPATHY

IgAN is most often diagnosed in persons 11–30 years of age but can be discovered in young children and older adults. Not all people with IgAN present in the same way. Only 15–20% of people present with visible blood in their urine (also termed macroscopic hematuria). This typically happens during an infection of the upper respiratory tract (such as a cold, sinus infection, or strep throat) or gastrointestinal tract (such as a stomach virus or inflammation of the colon). The urine may be pink, red, or brown but rarely has clumps of blood. During these episodes, people may have pain in their loins, flanks, or joints and, occasionally, mild fever. The visible blood in the urine may also be brought about by intense physical exercise in the absence of any apparent infection. The bleeding usually stops by itself after few days. If someone has an episode where they see blood in their urine due to IgAN, they often have similar episodes over the following years. In between these episodes of visible blood in the urine, microscopic hematuria (red blood cells

[RBCs] that can only be seen when the urine is inspected under a microscope) often persists and is reported as number of cells in a high-power-field view (RBC/HPF). Many adults with IgAN are diagnosed after a urinalysis taken at the time of a routine health checkup is evaluated as abnormal. Other adults, especially those younger than age 40, may be found to have kidney disease during evaluation for the cause of high blood pressure. Some of these patients have abnormal kidney function with an increased blood creatinine level. Presumably the IgAN has been present for years but without other signs or symptoms to lead to a medical evaluation. IgAN frequently causes protein to leak into the urine as well. A doctor will often check how much protein is leaking into the urine by testing the amount of all proteins in the urine—or just a specific protein called albumin, which accounts for about 40–70% of the protein in circulating blood. The measurement is reported as the protein–creatinine ratio or the albumin–creatinine ratio and is measured as milligrams per gram for a spot sample. Sometimes a 24-hour collection for protein is done and is measured as grams per day. The amount of protein that leaks into the urine can vary from person to person. Only in rare cases does that protein exceed three grams per day and lead to severe swelling due to retention of salt and water in tissues (edema). Tissue swelling due to proteinuria does occur in people with IgAN, though it is more common in children than adults. Acute kidney injury, defined as a significant increase in the level of creatinine in the blood over a span of less than three months, occurs in some patients with IgAN, and kidney function usually fully recovers after a few weeks. However, for some patients with acute kidney injury, the kidney biopsy shows severe inflammation and damage of the glomeruli. In this situation, intensive therapy to reduce the inflammation (for example, corticosteroids) is necessary.

MECHANISM OF DISEASE IN IGA NEPHROPATHY

The key to understanding the cause of IgAN is an appreciation of the unique structure of the IgA protein that accumulates in the glomeruli. This IgA is exclusively IgA1 (there are two types of IgA: IgA1 and IgA2). Its composition has less than a normal amount of a specific type of sugar, galactose, compared to the normal IgA1 in the circulating blood; this IgA is thus labelled galactose-deficient IgA1 (often abbreviated as Gd-IgA1).

Because its structure is different, the immune system of an IgAN patient sees it as a foreign object, much like bacteria or viruses, and attacks it. This starts an immune response where immune proteins attach to galactose-deficient

IgA1, forming small clusters that get physically stuck in the kidney's glomeruli, which leads to inflammation and eventual damage of those glomeruli. The current hypothesis of the development of IgAN is thought to be a four-step process (Figure 4), as follows:

Step 1: In patients with IgAN, the blood level of galactose-deficient IgA1 is higher than in healthy normal persons. They may have been born with an immune system that can create too much galactose-deficient IgA1.

Step 2: The immune system produces another antibody or immunoglobulin, in this case IgG, that recognizes the galactose-deficient IgA1 in the circulating blood as "foreign." This antibody is also called an autoantibody because it attacks a substance formed by a person's own body. This process of the body attacking itself is what defines IgAN as an autoimmune disease. These autoantibodies are possibly created when the immune system responds to a previous illness, then later mistakenly identifies the galactose-deficient IgA1 as a foreign invader and creates antibodies to fight it.

Step 3: When the IgA1 and the IgG autoantibodies bind together, complement component 3 (C3) also attaches, forming a complex cluster of immune proteins.

Step 4: As blood circulates through the kidney, some of these clusters get stuck and accumulate in the glomeruli to cause inflammation and kidney damage. This injury can lead to leakage of blood and protein into the urine. Continued injury may lead to scarring and reduce the capacity of the kidneys to filter waste products to clean the blood.

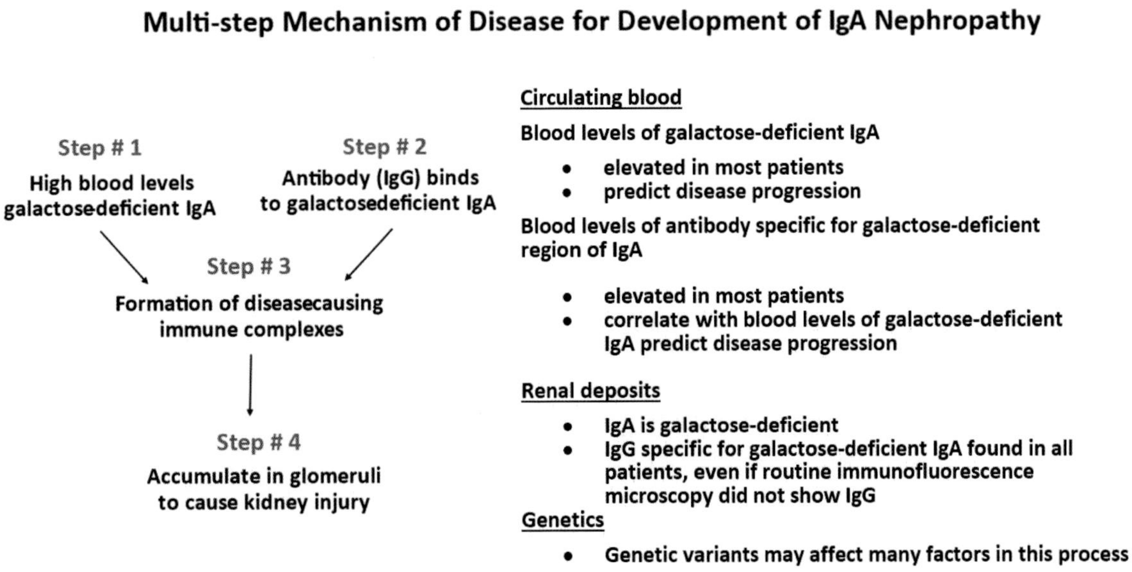

Figure 4.

Four-step proposed mechanism of disease for development of IgAN. High levels of galactose-deficient IgA1 in the circulating blood lead to production of an antibody (IgG) that recognizes the galactose-deficient IgA1 as "foreign." Some of this IgG binds to IgA1 to form immune clusters that may accumulate in the glomeruli to cause the kidney damage of IgAN. Additional details are shown on the right of the figure.

Genetic factors play an important role in the development of IgAN. Affected people who have one or more first-degree relatives (parent, sibling, child) also with IgAN are said to have familial IgAN. Those without an affected relative are said to have sporadic IgAN. Patients with either familial or sporadic IgAN may have variants of genes that increase the likelihood of having the disease. For example, the production of galactose-deficient IgA1 and the inflammatory response in the glomeruli due to the accumulation of the complexes with galactose-deficient IgA1 are influenced by several genetic factors. In fact, two genetic variants influence the production of galactose-deficient IgA1 so much that about 75% of IgAN patients and about 40% of their first-degree relatives have very high blood levels of galactose-deficient IgA1—evidence of it being an inheritable trait. As of late 2021, variants in 33 different portions of the human genome have been shown to affect the risk of having IgAN. The number of the genetic variants influences the age at which signs of kidney disease become evident. The higher the number of risk variants, the younger the age at diagnosis and the greater likelihood of abnormal kidney function. Furthermore, the number of these genetic variants that a person has accounts for some of the ethnic/racial differences in the frequency of IgAN: highest in Chinese, mid-range in whites, and lowest in Central Africans. The location of where the galactose-deficient IgA1 is produced has been a topic of increased interest in the last several years. Recent experimental studies suggest that galactose-deficient IgA1 is produced by cells that have been in "mucosal" tissues—for example, the cells lining the inside surfaces of the small intestine, colon, or tonsils. The IgA1 produced in these tissues protects us against infectious organisms and toxic materials in the environment. However, it is likely that some of these IgA1-producing cells leave the mucosal tissues to settle in the bone marrow. After relocation, the galactose-deficient IgA1 made by these cells can easily enter the circulating blood, where autoantibodies attach to form clusters that later accumulate in the glomeruli to cause IgAN. Currently, no single bacterium, virus, or environmental toxin has been found to commonly cause IgAN by irritating mucosal tissues.

PREDICTING KIDNEY OUTCOME

Since you were diagnosed with IgAN, you have probably been wondering what your future holds. Specifically, you're probably wondering if your kidney function will get worse over time and what treatments are available to help you. One prognostic factor is the amount of protein found in your urine. The separating point for adults, according to a 2007 study, appeared to be one gram (1000 milligrams) of proteinuria each day. People who have more than one gram per day of proteinuria tend to lose kidney function much more quickly than people with less proteinuria. Moreover, as the protein in the urine increases, the rate of loss of kidney function tends to speed up. However, reducing the amount of protein in the urine slows the rate of loss of kidney function. More recent studies indicate that the separating point is 0.5 gram (500 milligrams) of proteinuria per day. Thus, it is very important to reduce proteinuria to preserve kidney function. In 2009, an international group of nephrologists and pathologists discovered that the findings within a kidney biopsy also have predictive value, independent of clinical information such as proteinuria. These findings make up the MEST-C Oxford Classification tool used for prediction of future kidney function loss in adults with IgAN. A later study in 2014 showed that this tool was also valid in children with IgAN. In 2019 Dr. Sean Barbour and colleagues combined the MEST-C scores with standard clinical information at the time of kidney biopsy to develop the International IgA Nephropathy Prediction Tool to predict risk for substantial decline in eGFR in adults. A year later, the formula used to predict risk was adjusted so that a second version of this tool can be used to predict the risk for children. For a more detailed explanation of these tools, please refer to Appendix A.

CHRONIC KIDNEY DISEASE

Besides looking at the kidney biopsy or the amount of proteinuria, the easiest way to understand how much IgAN has affected a person's kidneys, is by looking at the stage of chronic kidney disease. A person is said to have chronic kidney disease if an abnormality of kidney function or structure is present for more than three months. Chronic kidney disease is broken down into five stages based on GFR and three groups based on albuminuria (Figure 5). As the filtration of the kidneys (GFR) decreases, the complications of chronic kidney disease usually increase because the kidneys aren't working as well. These complications can include high blood pressure, atherosclerosis (hardening of arterial blood vessels), salt and water buildup (increased blood pressure or fluid swelling in body tissues), challenges with bone health (low blood calcium and vitamin D levels and high blood phosphorus levels), and anemia (low hematocrit). Most IgAN patients with an eGFR of less than 30 mL/min/1.73 square meters body surface area progress to kidney failure and need dialysis or a kidney transplant.

Prognosis of CKD by GFR and albuminuria categories: KDIGO 2012

				description and range		
				A1	A2	A3
				Normal to mildly increased	Moderately increased	Severely increased
				<30 mg/g <3 mg/mmol	30–300 mg/g 3–30 mg/mmol	>300 mg/g >30 mg/mmol
GFR categories (ml/min/1.73 m²), description and range	G1	Normal or high	≥90			
	G2	Mildly decreased	60–89			
	G3a	Mildly to moderately decreased	45–59			
	G3b	Moderately to severely decreased	30–44			
	G4	Severely decreased	15–29			
	G5	Kidney failure	<15			

green, low risk (if no other markers of kidney disease, no CKD); yellow, moderately increased risk; orange, high risk; red, very high risk.

Figure 5.

Current chronic kidney disease (CKD) nomenclature (descriptions) used by Kidney Disease Improving Global Outcomes (KDIGO), based on GFR and amount of albumin in the urine (albuminuria). There are five groups/stages based on GFR and three groups based on albuminuria that impact the risk for development of kidney failure. Published in Kidney International (Supplement), volume 100, page S15, 2021.

TREATMENT

Recommendations and guidelines for treatment of patients with IgAN are included in the Kidney Disease Improving Global Outcomes (KDIGO) documents published periodically in Kidney International, a leading journal for the medical community caring for patients with kidney disease. The most recent guidelines for patients with glomerular kidney diseases, including IgAN, were published in October 2021. The central approach to treating IgAN focuses on control of blood pressure and proteinuria, treatment of high blood levels of triglycerides and cholesterol, correction of metabolic acidosis (low blood level of bicarbonate shown as CO2 on laboratory reports), sodium restriction to less than two grams per day with a heart-healthy diet, cessation of use of tobacco and nicotine products, weight control, and exercise as appropriate (Table 1).

Control of high blood pressure and proteinuria are extremely important. The target systolic blood pressure (the top number in the measurement) in most adults is about 120 mm Hg, while that in children is below the fiftieth percentile for their age, sex, and height. The initial treatment of high blood pressure should include an angiotensin converting enzyme inhibitor (ACEi) or angiotensin receptor blocker (ARB) because these drugs also reduce the damage of the glomeruli due to accumulation of IgA that causes proteinuria.

As control of proteinuria preserves long-term kidney function, proteinuria for adults that is greater than 500 milligrams per day and for children, greater than 200 milligrams per day (roughly, greater than 400 milligrams per 1.73 square meters body surface area per day, or greater than 200 milligrams per gram of creatinine) should be treated with an ACEi or ARB. The goal for adults is to maintain proteinuria at less than 500 milligrams per day; for children, at or under 200 milligrams per day (roughly at or under 400 milligrams per 1.73 square meters body surface area per day, or 200 milligrams per gram of creatinine). Because ACEi and ARB medications have serious potential side effects for a fetus, women considering pregnancy should discuss the implications of stopping this therapy with their doctor before conception.

Another option for adults with eGFR at or greater than 30 mL/min/1.73 square meters body surface area is a six-month course of high-dose corticosteroid therapy. The risk for significant side effects, particularly for patients with eGFR at or less than 50 mL/min/1.73 square meters body surface area, must be carefully considered. In special situations, such as acute kidney injury or a recent biopsy with extra cells in a crescent pattern around the glomerular tuft combined with a rising blood creatinine level, additional immunosuppression therapy may be appropriate.

Adults with proteinuria at greater than one gram per day despite optimized supportive care for three months should consider additional therapy available in a clinical trial (where newly available medications are evaluated). The number of trials has increased dramatically since 2018. Information about the trials, including the eligibility for participation, enrollment status, and treatment, is easily available at the ClinicalTrials.gov website of the National Institutes of Health. At the time of the preparation of this cookbook, several trials were nearing completion. You should talk with your nephrologist to discuss whether any newly approved medication may be appropriate for you.

The KDIGO guideline has limited recommendations for the diet of patients with chronic kidney diseases due to glomerular injury, such as IgAN. Dietary sodium restriction has been shown to improve blood pressure control and outcomes for kidney function. Additional recommendations for dietary approaches that are helpful for patients with chronic kidney disease are discussed elsewhere in this cookbook by Dr. Shusterman.

For children with proteinuria under one gram per day—or above one gram per gram creatinine, or with an M1 score in the Oxford Classification of the kidney biopsy—many pediatric nephrologists will treat with corticosteroids plus ACEi or ARB. Duration of therapy has not been established but is generally four weeks of 1-2 milligrams per kilogram body weight per day of oral prednisolone (or its equivalent) and then an alternate-day tapering schedule for four to six months.

For patients who progress to kidney failure, kidney transplantation is the best option for kidney replacement therapy. Because IgAN is due to a circulating factor (immune clusters with galactose-deficient IgA1), the disease often recurs in the new kidney. In fact, the frequency is as high as 50–70% at five years after transplantation. There is no therapy to prevent IgA from accumulating in the transplanted kidney, but inclusion of prednisone as one of the immunosuppressive medications and early use of ACEi or ARB appear to lessen the damage. Fortunately, most transplanted kidneys function well for years. inclusion of prednisone as one of the immunosuppressive medications and early use of ACEi or ARB appear to lessen the damage. Fortunately, most transplanted kidneys function well for years.

IGA VASCULITIS (ALSO KNOWN AS HENOCH–SCHOENLEIN PURPURA, OR HSP)

Previously termed Henoch–Schoenlein purpura (HSP), IgA vasculitis is an inflammation of the blood vessels due to accumulation of IgA. It affects children more commonly than adults. The accumulation of IgA in walls of the vessels causes leakage of blood into the nearby tissues. In skin, this process may cause raised red bumps (called purpura) that characteristically occur mostly below the waist. In the stomach or intestines, the inflammation may cause abdominal pain, and blood may enter the stool. Some patients develop ulcers in the skin, stomach, or intestines. Involvement in the joints may cause pain that affect several areas simultaneously before moving to other joints. The lungs and brain are only rarely affected. In nearly half of patients with IgA vasculitis, the kidneys are affected about four to six weeks after the appearance of the skin rash. A urinalysis usually shows hematuria and proteinuria. Adults progress to abnormal kidney function more often than children do. The findings on kidney biopsy are indistinguishable from those taken from IgAN patients. However, the Oxford Classification has not been validated for patients with IgA vasculitis with kidney involvement; nor is the IgAN Prediction Tool designed to predict kidney outcomes for these patients.

The KDIGO guideline includes recommendations for IgA vasculitis patients whose kidneys are affected. First off, the document recommends against the use of corticosteroids to prevent any kidney involvement. Treatment of the patients who develop kidney disease is like that for patients with IgAN. For patients who progress to kidney failure, transplantation is the optimal kidney replacement therapy. In some transplant recipients, IgA accumulates in the glomeruli of the new kidney in the pattern of IgAN, but involvement of the skin and other organs is uncommon.

SUPPORTIVE THERAPY IN IGA NEPHROPATHY	
THERAPY	**ACTIONS**
Control of Blood Pressure	• Most adults, target systolic blood pressure is 120 mm Hg • Children, target 24-hour systolic blood pressure is under fiftieth percentile for age, sex, and height by ambulatory blood pressure monitoring
Use of ACEi or ARB	• Maximally tolerated dose of ACEi or ARB
Lifestyle modifications	• Heart-healthy diet • Ideal body weight • Adequate physical activity • Cessation of use of tobacco and nicotine products • Limited alcohol consumption • Control of metabolic acidosis (low blood bicarbonate level) • Emotional health care
Reduce risk of heart and vascular disease	• Control of blood levels of lipids (triglycerides and cholesterol) ▪ Statins can be considered if age is over eight years ▪ Non-statin therapy • Anti-coagulation, review with doctor

TABLE 1 .

SLOWING KIDNEY DAMAGE THROUGH FOOD

By Dr. Blake Shusterman

When approached by the IgAN Foundation to contribute to this book, I was thrilled. It's an honor to write directly to all of you with IgA nephropathy (IgAN) as well as your friends, family, and loved ones. IgAN is a complex and varied illness, and people with IgAN have a wide spectrum of disease. You may have recently been diagnosed with IgAN with normal kidney function and no symptoms, you may have had IgAN for 30 years with chronic kidney disease, you may have IgAN that has progressed rapidly and led you to be near dialysis with swelling and difficult to control high blood pressure, or you may even be on dialysis or have had a kidney transplant.

I am writing to share good news for all of you.

No matter where you are on your IgAN journey, choosing the right foods and paying close attention to your diet can help you. It can lead to lower blood pressure, slow the decline of kidney function, help keep you out of the hospital, and lower the protein in your urine. This book is designed to help you do all of that.

When I first started caring for people with IgAN more than ten years ago, I was struck by the lack of treatment options we, nephrologists, had to help people to slow down their kidney disease and keep them off dialysis. Though many improvements have been made over the last decade, and more improvements are visible on the horizon, you may have encountered the same reality: There is no definitive treatment for IgAN. For you or your family member, that realization may bring a feeling that your kidney disease is somewhat out of your control.

People throughout the spectrum of kidney disease feel that way, leaving doctors and patients feeling helpless after this difficult diagnosis. Faced with this reality, I started researching non-medication treatment options to see if there was any advice I could give people to help them take charge of their health and make a noticeable difference in the severity of their kidney disease. And fortunately, being a lover of good food and cooking, I stumbled across a wealth of data suggesting that dietary changes can play a large role in the management of kidney disease and IgAN.

As I studied more and worked to teach my patients—and you—how to eat healthier and choose foods that fit their illnesses, I realized this strategy gave them confidence. They developed a sensation that control of their kidney disease was within their reach. I decided to dedicate my time to teaching people how to use food to manage their kidney disease, developed an online persona called the Cooking Doc, and wrote a book called The Cooking Doc's Kidney-Healthy Cooking: A Modern 10-Step Guide to Preventing and Managing Kidney Disease. In this chapter I will share much of what I know and relate it directly to IgAN.

Is diet going to cure your IgAN or definitively keep you off of dialysis? Certainly not. Diet is a helpful tool, but it is not a magical treatment or miracle cure. It is to be used together with other treatments. The course of IgAN often lasts many years. You may be diagnosed with the disease in your teens or twenties and have to manage the consequences of the disease for the next fifty years or longer. That means you will need to maintain a healthy diet for decades.

What are the keys to successfully sticking with a long-term diet? Make the food tasty, create a lifestyle that allows you to cook meals at home, and develop a culture in your household that prioritizes the health and wellness of your kidneys.The recipes in this book are my kind of recipes. They are fresh, flavorful, creative, accessible to the home cook, and absolutely delicious.

HOW KIDNEYS REACT TO FOOD

Kidneys are responsible for processing many of the waste products that your body produces during the day. A large amount of these waste products comes from the foods you eat. Whether you eat a hamburger, fries, and a coke, or quinoa with broccoli, tofu, and kombucha, that food gets broken down in the gastrointestinal (GI) tract and absorbed into your body. It then flows through the blood to the kidneys, where they determine which products of that food need to be returned to the body to help nurture it, and which should be excreted in the urine. Sometimes the work is easy for the kidneys, while other times they work extra hard to process these products.

The diet for people with IgAN or any type of kidney disease can be broken down into two parts. The first part is foods and eating patterns that will protect your kidneys, keep your kidney disease from getting worse, and help manage your blood pressure. The second part comes into play if your kidney disease gets worse. As the kidneys lose their ability to filter your blood and maintain balance (also known as homeostasis)—and this is measured in your blood tests through things like blood urea nitrogen (BUN), creatinine, potassium, bicarbonate, phosphorus, and others—it becomes more important to eat foods that your kidneys can easily process and allow them to maintain that balance even in their damaged state.

While the information in this book discusses a general overview of how the body and the kidneys react to these things, the most effective and best diet for someone with kidney disease is individualized using the help of a kidney dietitian.

THERE IS NO ONE-SIZE-FITS-ALL DIET FOR PEOPLE WITH IGA NEPHROPATHY.

When you went to see your doctor last time for an IgAN follow-up, you may have been told you have chronic kidney disease (CKD), and your specific stage. Your stage of kidney disease does not necessarily tell you exactly how to eat to protect your kidneys, and that's why everyone with kidney disease needs the help of a dietitian. Knowing the stage of your kidney disease may give you a broad guidance as to what you need to eat; for instance, if I see two people with stage IV CKD from IgAN, certain things will surely be the same in their diet. A closer look at their needs, though, may show that they have significantly different restrictions on their potassium or phosphorus intake. How much of each you can safely eat depends on a lot of things—from your estimated glomerular filtration rate (eGFR), to whether or not you have diabetes, to the level of potassium and phosphorus in your blood, to the medications you take.

The bottom line is, try to find a dietitian to work with if you have questions or need specific information about your nutritional needs. Every choice you make during the day makes an impact on your kidney disease. The more you know, the more you pay attention and the more you cook at home, the better you'll be able to help manage your kidney disease. Not only that, but the food you choose to eat can help you manage your blood pressure, keep your swelling down, and make you feel better as you go about your day-to-day activities.

SODIUM

Let's talk about salt and sodium.

When you eat foods that contain a lot of salt, your kidneys are in charge of getting rid of the extra. When they can't get rid of the salt, they hold onto it; and then they hold on to extra water as well, because water will follow that salt. That extra salt and extra water can make blood pressure worse, and contribute to worsening protein in your urine and worsening swelling, or fluid buildup, in your legs. As your kidney function gets worse, the kidneys may become even more sensitive to that extra salt.

As the Cooking Doc, I've counseled many people about the benefits of a low-sodium diet and I have seen some amazing results. By learning to cook at home, and cooking lower-sodium foods, my patients become better chefs. Their diet and their taste buds change from craving high-sodium, high-fat, high-sugar, high-carbohydrate foods to seeking out fresh fruits and vegetables, herbs like cilantro and basil, citrus like lemon and lime—and it brings out their curiosity in eating. Are you ready to find that same inspiration?

If you have been to the doctor, you've probably heard "eat a low-sodium diet" as the generic advice out there. You've probably also been told the basics: 70% or more of the sodium in the diet of people in the United States comes from processed foods and restaurant foods. If you have already worked on eliminating these two sources of sodium, you are probably cooking a majority of your meals at home and have already changed your taste buds to enjoy the flavors of fresh and frozen herbs, citrus, and lower-sodium meals. If you are just starting out, though, and eating a majority of your meals at restaurants or by putting prepackaged food in the microwave, I have good news and bad news for you. The good news is that it's easy to locate the extra sodium in your diet and make a few easy and meaningful changes. The bad news is that your taste buds are likely so used to high-sodium foods that you will think foods with less sodium taste bland when you start out making these changes.

A lower-sodium diet can benefit people with IgAN in many ways. It can lower the amount of protein in your urine, help you control your blood pressure, and help you keep fluid from building up inside your body.

A low-sodium diet means consuming less than 2,300 milligrams of sodium each day, which is slightly less than the 2,325 milligrams of sodium in one teaspoon of salt. In the United States, the average daily sodium intake is 3,400 milligrams. That's 1,100 mg more than the recommendation—or approximately one tablespoon of soy sauce, half a teaspoon of table salt, a medium-large pickle, three ounces of sliced ham, or two hot dogs. So, if you're not actively paying attention to how much sodium you're eating, you're likely eating more than recommended for a person with IgAN.

I recommend you start by identifying the largest sources of sodium in your diet. Once you have identified the part or parts of your diet that give you the most sodium, you can think about how you can lower that intake.

How many meals do you eat out at restaurants during a week?	Each restaurant meal has more sodium than you need. Though it can be difficult to limit your sodium when you are eating out, try a few easy tips: ask for all sauces on the side, use oil/vinegar on salads instead of salad dressing, avoid the fried foods and dips, and skip the pre-meal bread.
How many times do you eat fast food in a week?	Cut out as many of these instances as possible. It is nearly impossible to eat a low-sodium meal when at a fast food restaurant.
Does your diet consist of frozen meals or canned or boxed foods? If so, do you ever read the nutrition label on these foods to see how much sodium they contain?	Learn to read nutrition labels and choose options that are low or no sodium. Choose frozen vegetables instead of canned vegetables. If making boxed meals, use your own no-sodium seasoning instead of the spice pack that comes with it.
Do you snack on chips, pretzels, or crackers?	Try veggies and fruit instead.
Are you a lover or frequent consumer of processed meats like salami, bologna, and pepperoni or sliced deli meats like turkey, ham, or roast beef?	Choose no-sodium versions from the deli counter or create your own chicken and turkey at home by roasting turkey or chicken breasts and slicing them up to use during the week.
Do you like your foods covered in sauces such as ketchup, barbeque sauce, or jarred salsa?	Find no-sodium versions or use only a teaspoon.
Is your pantry and refrigerator filled with foods like pickles and olives to eat alongside your meals?	Leave them at the grocery store. These high-sodium snacks add up quickly.
Do you salt your food before you taste it?	Taste your food and then put the salt in your hand before you add it to taste. Use only a tiny bit.

The next step is learning to create flavors without using a lot of salt. One of my favorite recipes in this book, the Spring Pesto Salad, provides a great example of ways to create flavor without salt. Chef Emma uses basil, parsley, garlic, and lemon to develop a dish that doesn't need a lot of salt to still pop with flavor.

POTASSIUM

When you got your diagnosis of IgAN and looked up a kidney-friendly diet, did you immediately start cutting out high-potassium foods? If you did, you're not alone. Many people are under the impression that a low-potassium diet is recommended for people with kidney disease, but this isn't the case for many especially if you have only recently been diagnosed with IgAN or if you have stage I–III CKD.

Here's the complicated truth.

A high-potassium diet is beneficial for you until your kidney disease reaches a certain point, and then you may need to switch to a diet that is lower in potassium. In some people, the need for a low-potassium diet may happen when their kidneys are functioning at 30%, while others—for reasons we don't completely understand—may never reach a point where they need to limit their dietary potassium. These nuances have led to some confusion, because recommendations often get lumped into an incorrect one-size-fits-all recommendation: "Everyone with kidney disease needs to limit their potassium." That is not the truth.

For most people, a high-potassium diet actually provides many health benefits. If your kidneys are processing potassium correctly, a high-potassium diet can lower your risk of developing a stroke and help you manage your blood pressure. That's because the kidneys can use that extra potassium to get rid of extra sodium in the body. This helps the body retain less water, thus lowering blood pressure. There are also other complex reasons why potassium helps lower blood pressure, but we don't understand them fully at this time.

The benefits of a high-potassium diet extend even farther. High-potassium foods add to the alkalinity of your diet, reduce your risk of kidney stones, and provide you with added fiber and micronutrients. If the kidneys are working at full strength, they can handle about as much potassium as you can eat, but problems occur when the kidneys have difficulty filtering blood and can't process extra potassium in the diet. Once kidney function dips to a eGFR below 30 milliliters per minute (approximately 30% function)—and this is what occurs in stages IV and V CKD—things change for some people. At that point, the kidneys may have trouble filtering potassium, and potassium can build up in the blood. While this often causes people to need to limit the potassium in their diet, it's important to note that other things such as medications, high blood sugars, and high blood acid levels can raise the blood potassium, and don't necessarily have much to do with how much potassium you are eating. For example, the primary treatment for many people with IgAN includes a class of medications called angiotensin receptor blockers (ARBs) or angiotensin converting enzyme inhibitors (ACEi). Both of these medications can raise the potassium in your blood without you ever changing how much potassium is in your diet. In these circumstances, you will need to discuss with your doctor the best way to lower the potassium in your blood and see if that includes limiting potassium in your diet, adjusting your current medication, or adding a new medication. Remember that you should never make adjustments in your medications without first speaking to your physician.

We nephrologists are actually still learning exactly how the potassium in a person's diet raises or lowers the potassium in your blood. While we figure this out, it's important to speak with your doctor or dietitian to see if you need to limit your dietary potassium.

This book offers a mixture of high-potassium and low-potassium dishes. Because there aren't any meat-containing recipes in this book, the potassium all comes through vegetables, fruits, and grains. These foods contain potassium but also contain fiber, an ingredient missing from the diet of many people. This fiber leads to more regular bowel movements and can actually help your body process extra dietary potassium because you can also lose potassium in your stool. (I know this is a book about food, so gross!—but understanding how your body gets rid of potassium through urine and stool will help you figure out how to best manage your diet.)

I'd also like to mention meat as well. Though it gets ignored in many articles about potassium, meat actually contains a significant amount of it. For example, did you know that a cup of chicken breast has about as much potassium as a medium tomato? But, has anyone ever told you to eat less chicken to manage your potassium? I'll bet they never have. It seems like they always tell you to cut out your tomatoes instead.

The most important thing to know about dietary potassium and IgAN is, there is not one recommendation that applies to everyone with kidney disease. Consult with a dietitian, review your labs, and gain the insight as to how much potassium is right for you.

PROTEIN

Your body needs protein to survive. The protein that you eat gets broken down in the digestive tract and goes on to serve as the building blocks of the hormones that circulate in the body and to help build muscle mass. In the United States, the average person's diet already exceeds the protein intake that the body needs to function properly. That means our diet contains more protein than we actually need. Much of that protein comes from meat.Even though this protein intake exceeds the minimum amount the body needs to thrive, people with normal kidney function usually don't have a problem with the extra protein. Things change if you have been diagnosed with IgAN and have protein in your urine or have developed CKD. In that case, consuming more protein than your body needs or eating too much animal protein may cause trouble.

Scientists are still working to determine the exact mechanisms by which extra protein affects the kidneys. The most recent hypotheses revolve around the idea that eating too much protein, especially if it is animal protein, leads to extra pressure inside the kidneys and causes the tiny filters inside the kidney to over-filter, or hyper-filter. This response may cause scars to form in the filters (the glomeruli) of the kidneys. When these filters develop scars, the kidneys' capacity to filter the blood is reduced, and kidney function may decline. One of the primary goals of getting your diet right for your kidneys - consuming the right kinds of foods in the right amounts - is to keep as many of the kidneys' filters working for as long as possible.

Based on the most recent recommendations and my evaluation of the literature, the optimal protein intake for people with IgAN is 0.25 to 0.35 g/lb/d (that means 0.35 grams of protein for each pound of body weight each day, or, as an example, a 150-pound-person targeting 52.5 grams of protein each day), and most of that protein should come from plants. This recommendation gets more important as your kidney function worsens. For example, a strict protein limit provides more benefit for people with stage V CKD as compared to people with stage III CKD. That means that if you have stage III CKD, your focus should be on watching your sodium intake, eating the right amount of potassium, and substituting plant proteins for animal proteins, and not on calculating your exact daily protein needs.

All of the recipes inside this book contain only plant protein. Years ago, there was a belief that you couldn't get all the nutrients you needed from plant protein, but that's only true if you're getting all of your plant protein from one source, such as beans. However, there are many ways to get plant-based protein in your diet. By choosing a variety of sources for your protein—such as a mixture of beans, whole grains, seeds, lentils, nuts, and tofu—you can ensure you get the right kinds of protein to keep your body healthy.

One final thought before we leave the protein section. Just because all of the recipes in this book are plant-based, doesn't mean you can't include some animal protein in your diet. For many people, the convenience of meat—both the ease of cooking and buying it, the familiarity of you and your family with the flavors, and the way it fits seamlessly into many of our favorite recipes—make it difficult to give up. So, if you are not interested in giving up all meat or don't know how to start eating plant based, never fear. Here are a few suggestions for those of you who want more of a plant-based diet instead of a vegan diet. A plant-based diet is a diet focused on including plants as a part of your meals but does not necessarily mean you never eat meat.

- Eat meat only one time each day. Choose chicken or fish instead of beef or pork.
- Pick one day of the week and make it totally plant based.
- When eating meat, eat only three to four ounces, or pick a serving size that fits in the palm of your hand.

Use spices that you are used to cooking with, are low sodium, and contain flavors that you enjoy. For example, you could add a few ounces of shredded home-cooked chicken breast to the Burrito Bowl recipe.

PHOSPHORUS

Unless you have stage V CKD or are on dialysis, you probably don't have to worry about limiting the phosphorus in your diet. Good news, right?

Phosphorus is an element that can build up in your blood if you have CKD, but it usually only happens when kidney function falls below 20%.

Ready for more good news about phosphorus?

The biggest sources of easily absorbable phosphorus in the diet are dairy products, processed foods, and meat. None of these are found in the recipes in this book. So, if you are eating delicious food like the dishes presented here, you won't have to worry about how much phosphorus is in the food that you eat. The phosphorus in plant-based foods is not as readily absorbed as the phosphorus in food additives, animal protein, and dairy products. Those are the biggest sources of phosphorus to be concerned about. So, if you were told by your doctor to limit phosphorus, first look towards cutting out processed foods and lowering your intake of dairy products and animal proteins.

If you do find yourself at the store buying already prepared foods, look for the four-letter word phos hidden in the ingredient lists and know that those foods have extra phosphorus that is easily absorbed into your body.

HYDRATION

This section may surprise you. When most of us think about keeping kidneys healthy, we think about keeping the kidneys hydrated. Hydrated kidneys are happy kidneys. When the body has enough water, the kidneys are able to filter to the best of their abilities. They can also keep the electrolytes balanced and the waste products removed in the urine. While it seems intuitive, then, that you should drink a lot of water throughout the day to keep your kidneys happy, it's not exactly how the body works.

Your body has a complex system that keeps you hydrated. The leading driver to keep you hydrated is your thirst. When your body gets low on fluid, you get thirsty. That thirst drives you to grab a drink, and hydrate until your body is fully rehydrated. Because our bodies are complex systems, there is no magic to drinking eight eight-ounce glasses of water each day.

Unless you are sick with nausea, vomiting, or infection, out in the hot weather, or playing an active sport, you will probably be able to keep your kidneys happy and hydrated by reaching for a water bottle when you get thirsty, and not focusing on drinking a specific amount of water each day.

It's also important to know that foods play a large role in keeping you hydrated as well. Many foods are composed of more than 50% water; so your body will digest these foods and use the water in them to keep the kidneys working well.

There is one catch in all of this.

When many people get thirsty, they don't reach for water. They reach, instead, for a sugary beverage such as soda or juice. While those drinks will certainly help to keep you hydrated, their extra calories can put you at higher risk for obesity, high blood pressure, and diabetes—all of which can complicate a diagnosis of IgAN or CKD.

ANTI-INFLAMMATORY DIET

IgAN happens when a protein called IgA, which is typically part of the immune system, builds up in a part of the kidney that does the filtering. While it is not clear exactly what triggers this event, in many ways IgAN is an autoimmune disease because IgA attacks and causes damage to your kidneys rather than doing its job of protecting the body from infection.

There has been ongoing research to determine whether the foods you eat can either contribute to the inflammation that occurs with autoimmune disease or help prevent the inflammation from occurring. And, while we are still learning which foods cause inflammation and contribute to chronic disease, certain suggestive patterns have emerged.

Luckily for all of you, the foods that may increase inflammation are all avoided in this book. Certain diets such as the DASH diet, the Mediterranean diet, and a vegan diet have all been postulated to reduce inflammation. If you are interested in these diets but don't know much about them, you can find many descriptions of them on the web or in my book. All of the recipes in this book fit into these categories.

Moreover, and more importantly, many of the possibly inflammatory foods can be avoided by following a few easy rules:

- Limit or avoid fried foods
- Drink fewer or avoid sweetened beverages such as soda, juice, and sweet tea
- Stay away from refined carbohydrates such as white bread, rice, pasta, pretzels, etc.
- Avoid processed meats like hot dogs, sausage, bologna, and bacon
- Monitor your intake of saturated fats

The recipes in this book also avoid gluten. There is currently not enough research to suggest that eating gluten will worsen IgAN, and there is no study to suggest that avoiding gluten will help people with IgAN maintain their kidney function. There are suggestions of a link between gluten and IgAN in mice, but until that link is established in humans, there isn't a need to avoid all gluten when trying to eat a diet that will help you manage your IgAN.

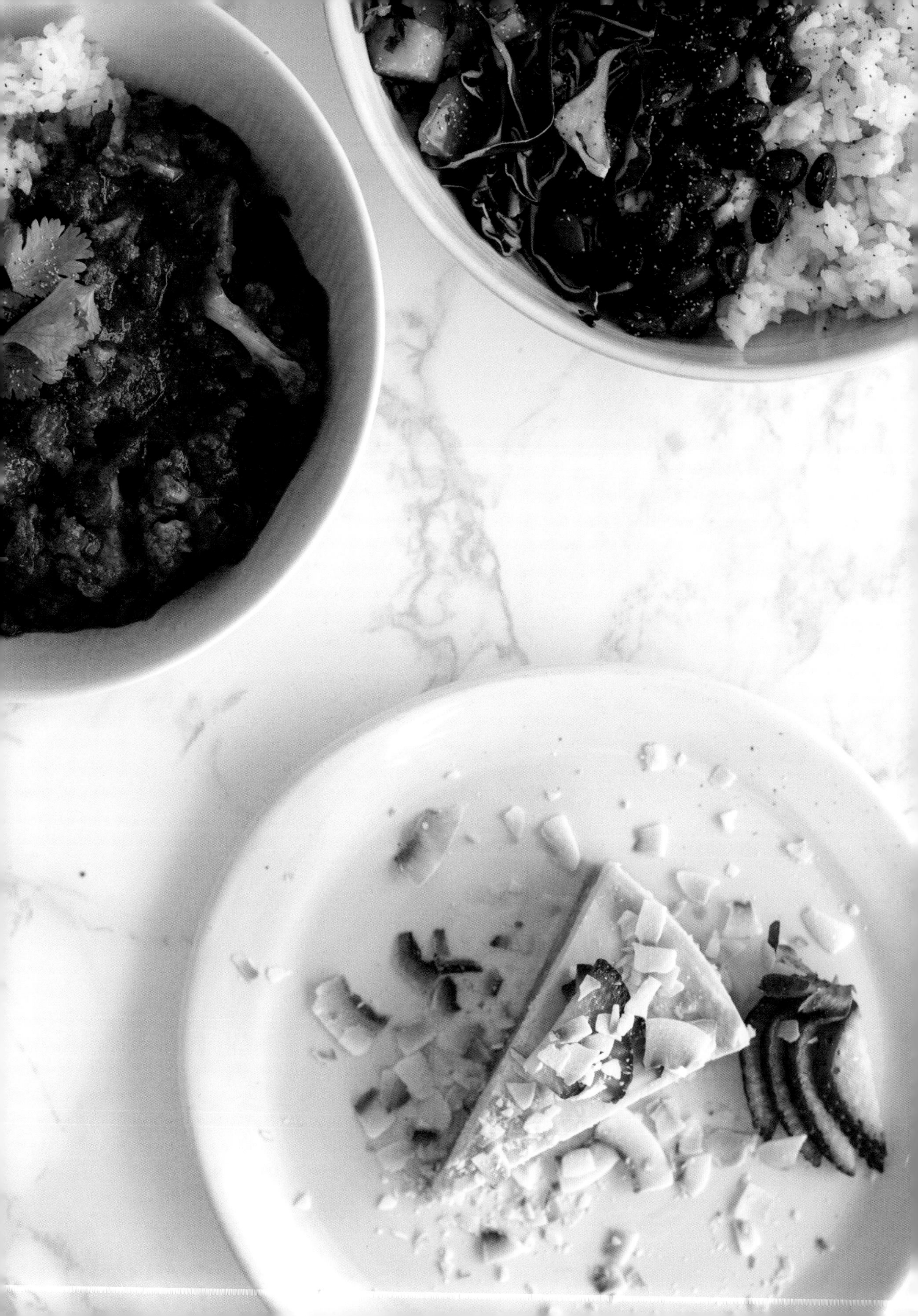

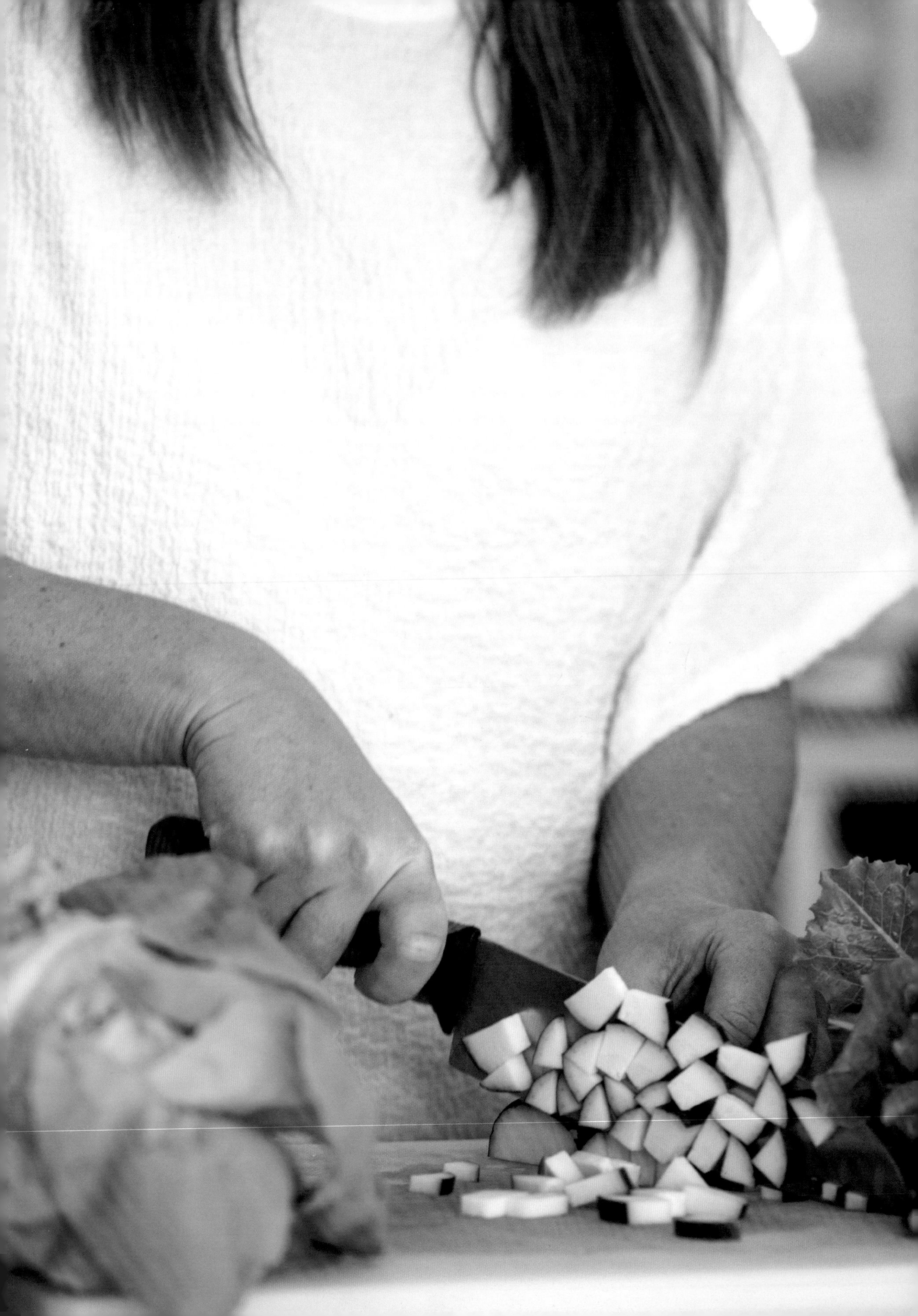

IgAN RECIPES

Hey there, IgAN warriors - it's Emma here. I hope you're ready get crafty in the kitchen and try out these plant-based recipes that were created with you in mind! No matter what your reason was for purchasing this cookbook, I hope that these recipes help kick-start a lifestyle change that serves your body well. Just remember, our bodies can do miraculous things when we give them the fuel and the care they deserve. Happy cooking! :)

Xo,
Emma

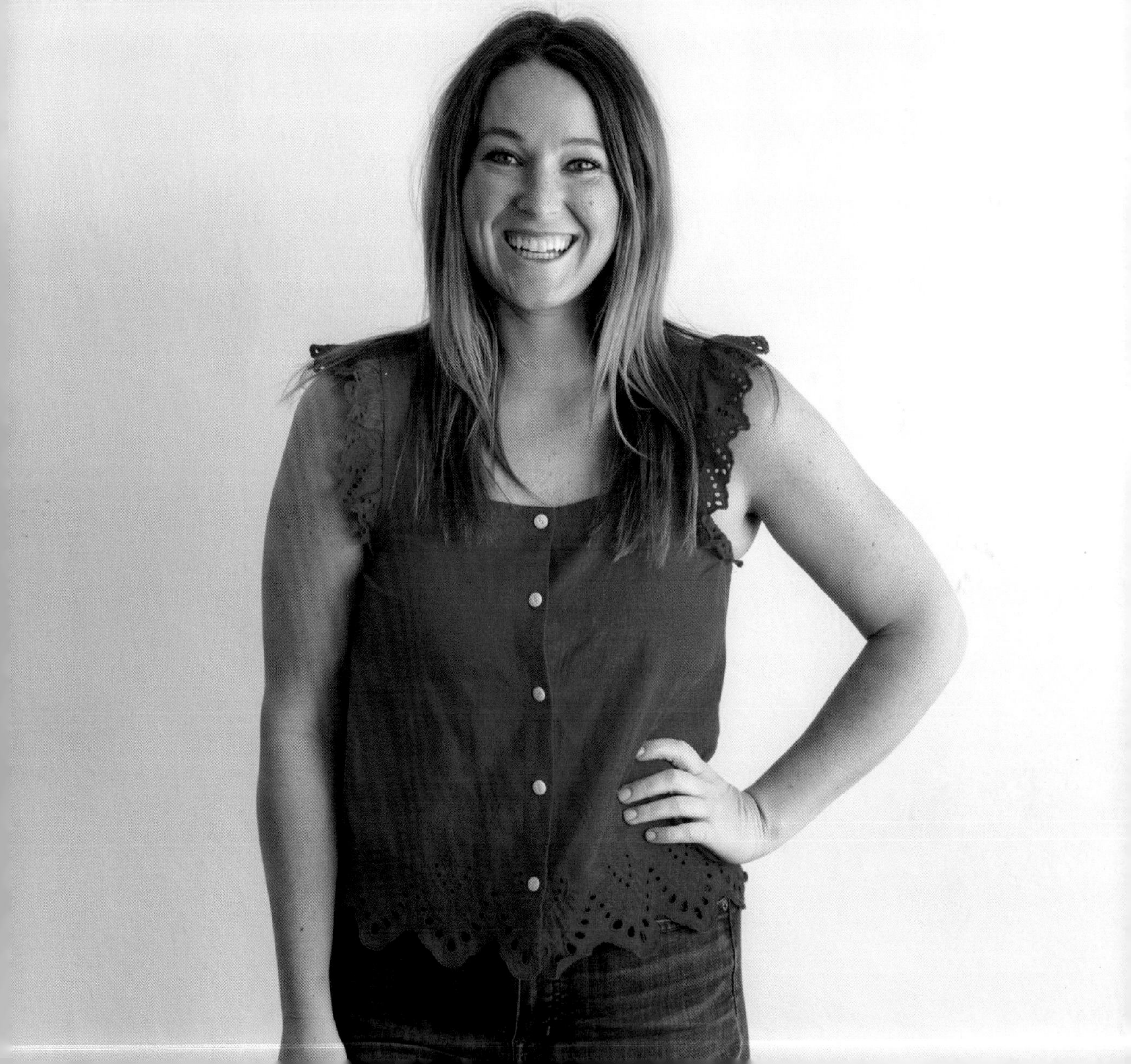

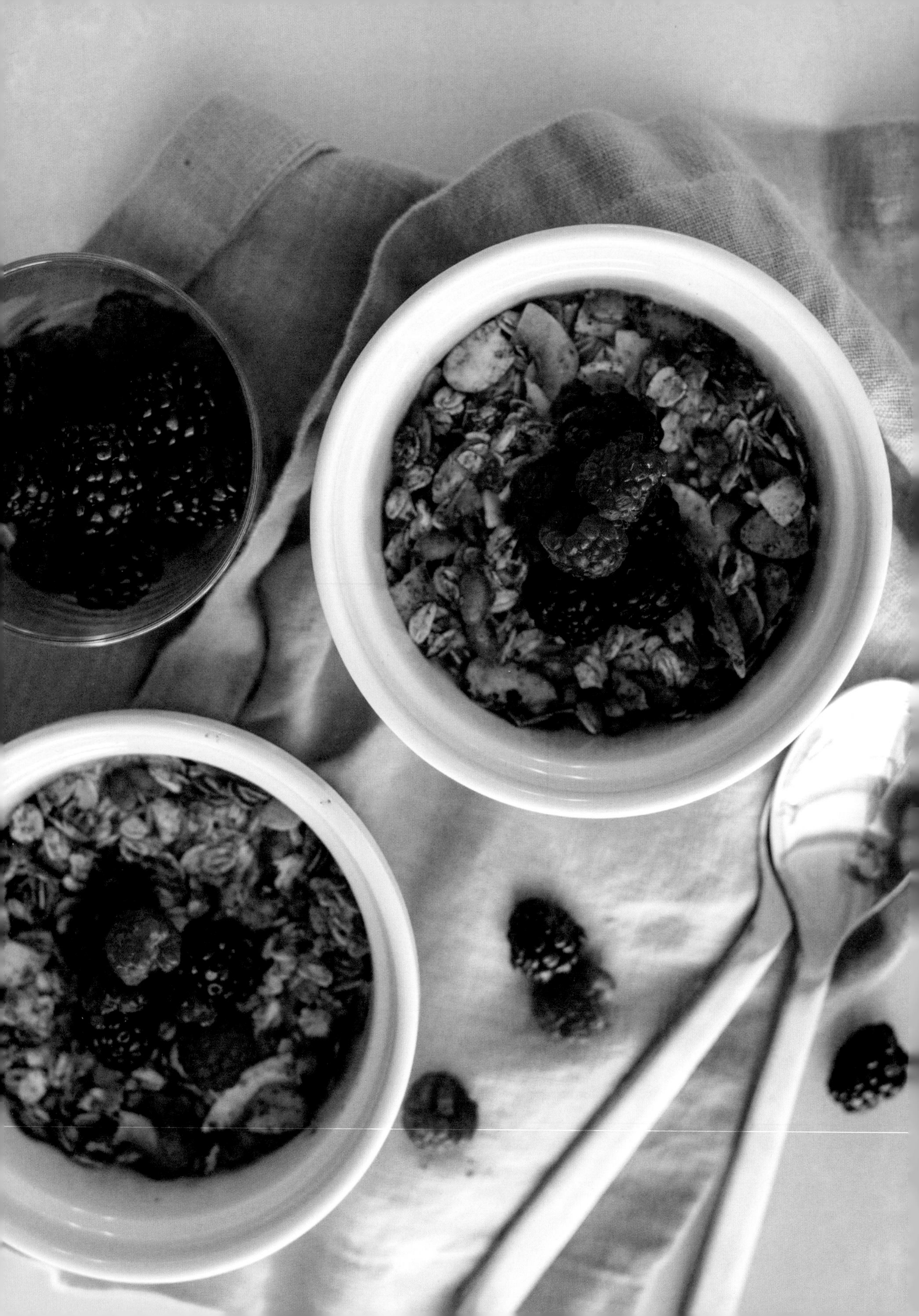

BREAKFAST

Berry-Green Smoothie

DAIRY-FREE | GLUTEN-FREE | NUT-FREE | VEGAN | VEGETARIAN

SERVES 1

Ingredients

½ cup frozen blueberries
½ cup frozen pineapple
½ cup frozen mango
1 cup fresh kale
1 inch of fresh ginger root
½ cup orange juice
½ cup water

Optional Superfoods

1Tbsp chia seeds
1Tbsp hemp seeds

Directions

1. Blend all ingredients on high in a blender until smooth and creamy. Depending on your blender, you may have to add additional liquid to blend. Serve immediately.

NEEDING LOWER POTASSIUM?
Substitute non-dairy milk for orange juice and arugula for kale.

KCALS 220 | CARBOHYDRATE 43 G | PROTEIN 6 G | FAT 5 G | SATURATED 5 G
SODIUM 47 MG | POTASSIUM 597 MG | FIBER 11 G | CALCIUM 275 MG
PHOSPHORUS 169 MG | IRON 3 MG

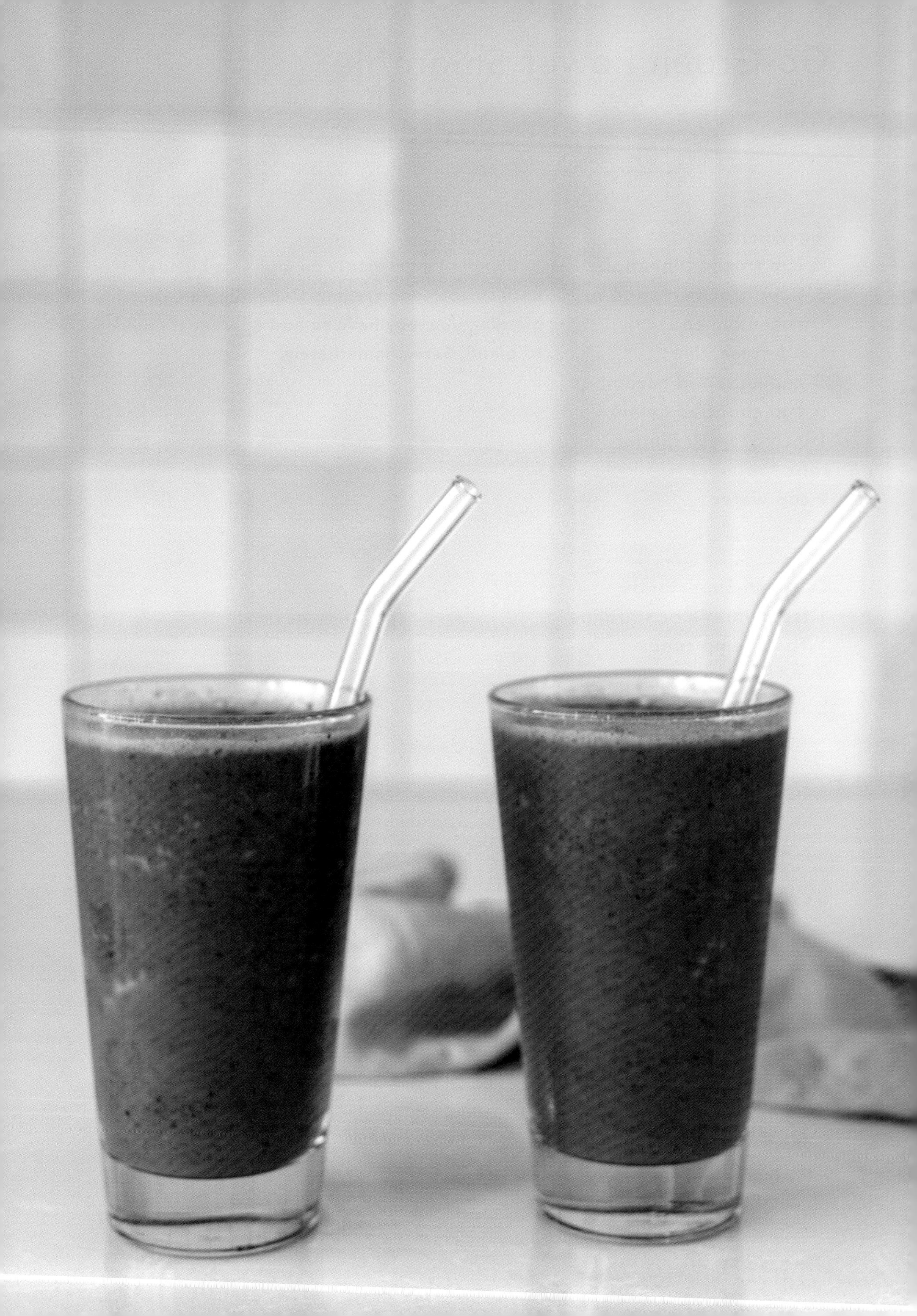

Go-Green Power Smoothie

DAIRY-FREE | GLUTEN-FREE | NUT-FREE | VEGAN | VEGETARIAN

SERVES 1

Ingredients

½ cup frozen pineapple
3/4 cup frozen mango or
1 frozen banana
1 cup fresh kale
¼ cup chopped cucumber
¼ cup chopped celery
1 inch of fresh ginger
root **optional*
1 cup water

Optional Superfoods

1 tsp chlorella or spirulina
1 Tbsp hemp seeds

Directions

1. Blend all ingredients on high in a blender until smooth and creamy. Depending on your blender, you may have to add additional liquid to blend. Serve immediately.

NEEDING LOWER POTASSIUM?
Substitute arugula for kale.

KCALS 174 | CARBOHYDRATE 30 G | PROTEIN 6 G | FAT 6 G | SATURATED FAT 1 G
SODIUM 43 MG | POTASSIUM 432 MG | FIBER 5 G | CALCIUM 91 MG
PHOSPHORUS 200 MG | IRON 2 MG

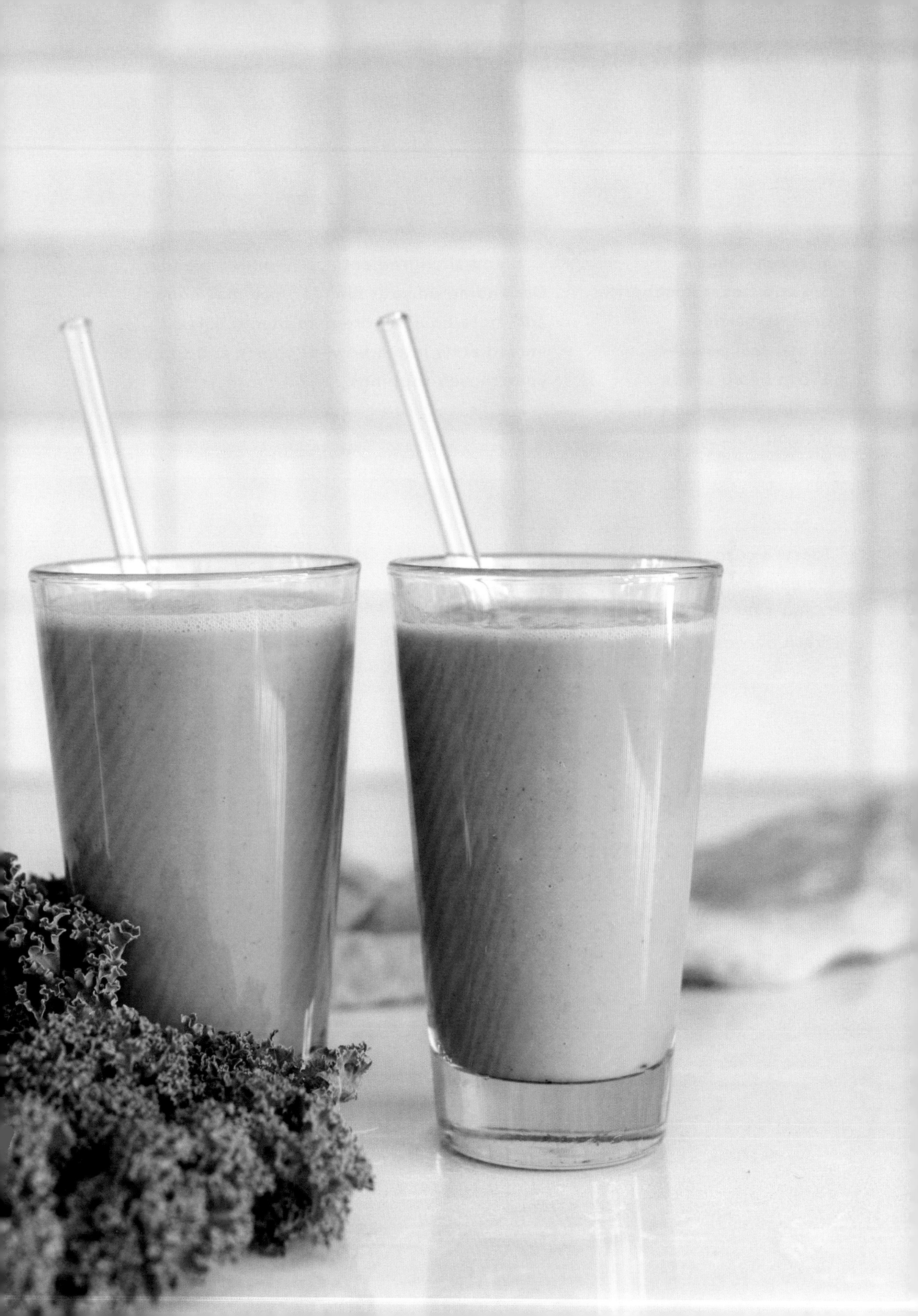

Acai Smoothie Bowl

DAIRY-FREE | GLUTEN-FREE | VEGAN | VEGETARIAN

SERVES 1

Ingredients

1 frozen banana
3/4 cup frozen blueberries or strawberries
1Tbsp acai powder
1Tbsp hemp seeds
½ cup orange juice or almond milk

Toppings

Toasted coconut flakes
Homemade granola (page 117)
Fresh berries

Directions

1. Blend all ingredients on high in a blender. Depending on your blender, you may need to add more liquid in order to blend. Serve immediately into a bowl of choice and top with your chosen toppings.

KCALS 332 | CARBOHYDRATE 46 G | PROTEIN 8 G | FAT 14 G | SATURATED FAT 1 G
SODIUM 165 MG | POTASSIUM 447 MG | FIBER 11 G | CALCIUM 183 MG
PHOSPHORUS 204 MG | IRON 3 MG

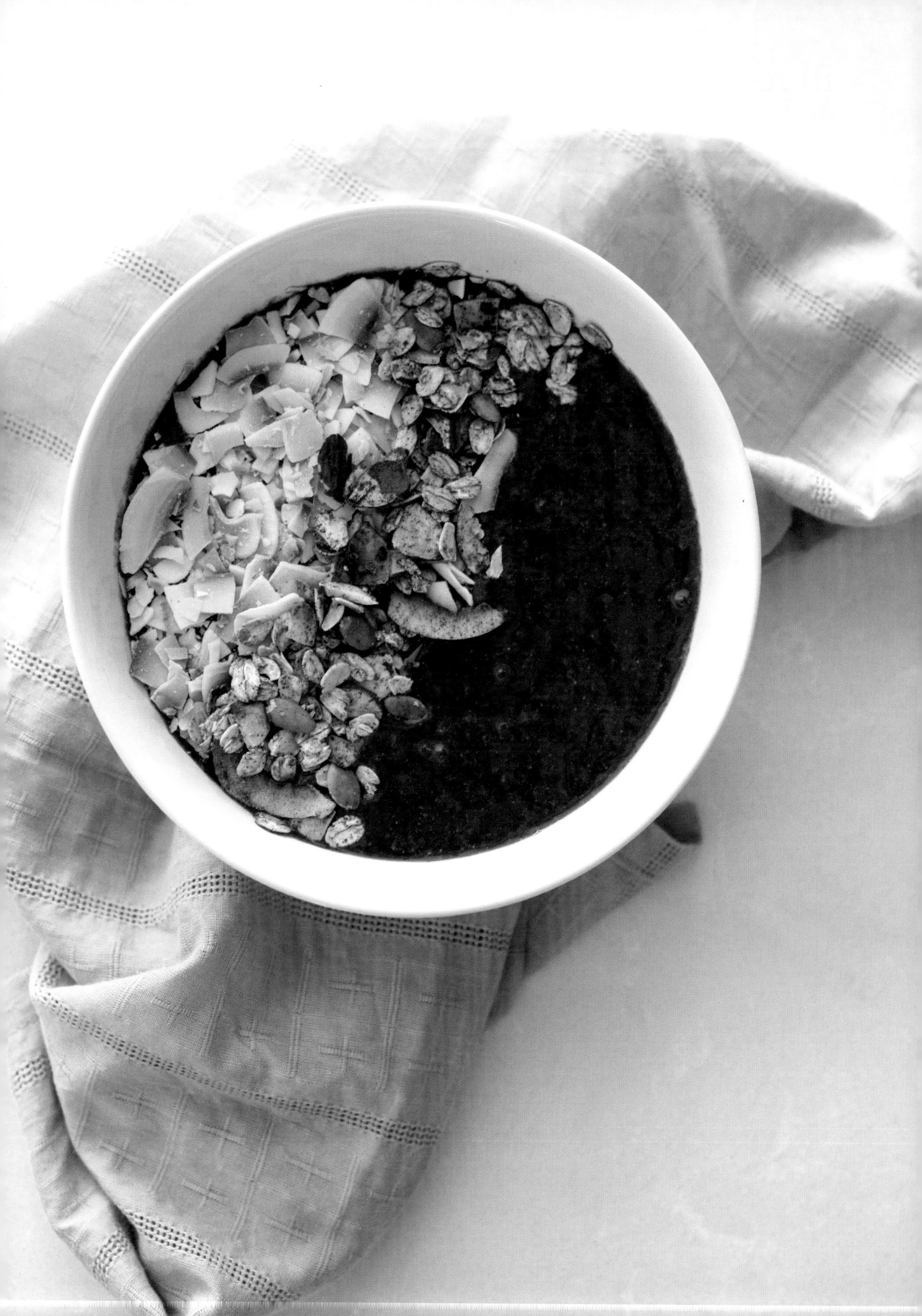

Blueberry Breakfast Muffins

DAIRY-FREE | GLUTEN-FREE | VEGAN | VEGETARIAN

SERVES 12

Ingredients

1 1/2 cups oat flour
3/4 cup almond flour
1 tsp baking powder
3/4 tsp baking soda
1/2 tsp sea salt
1 Tbsp ground flaxseed
1 cup applesauce
1/4 cup melted coconut oil
1/4 cup pure maple syrup
1 1/2 tsp vanilla extract
3/4 cup frozen blueberries

Directions

1. Preheat oven to 350F.
2. Add all dry ingredients to a bowl and whisk to combine.
3. Add all wet ingredients, except for the blueberries, to the dry mixture and mix well until thoroughly combined.
4. Add frozen blueberries and fold in lightly.
5. Scoop muffin mixture into silicone mold or muffin tins.
6. Bake for 12-15 minutes or until tops are lightly golden.

KCALS 176 | CARBOHYDRATE 20 G | PROTEIN 4 G | FAT 10 G | SATURATED FAT 4 G
SODIUM 205 MG | POTASSIUM 101 MG | FIBER 2 G | CALCIUM 54 MG
PHOSPHORUS 83 MG | IRON 1 MG

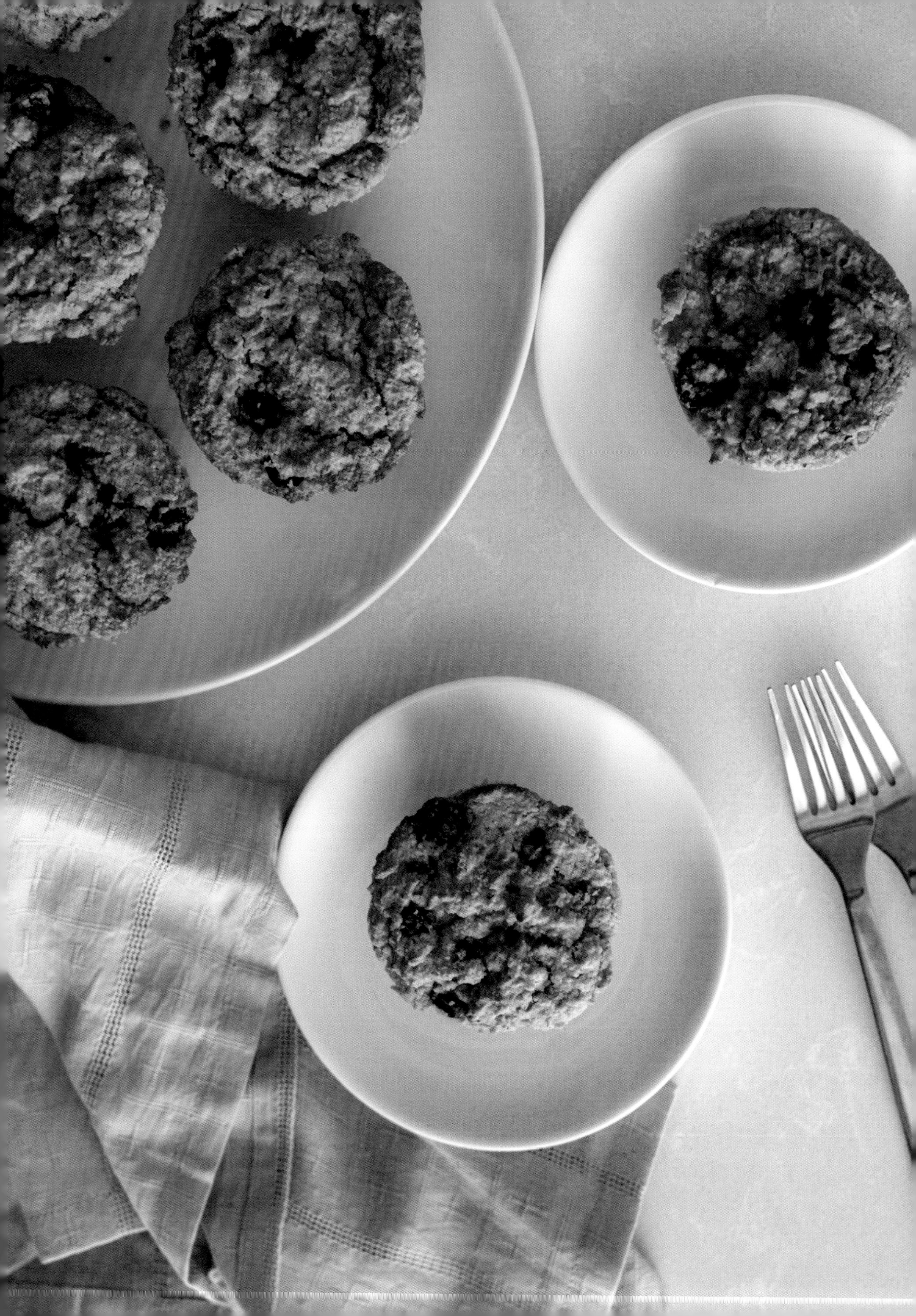

Apple Cinnamon Oatmeal

DAIRY-FREE | GLUTEN-FREE | NUT-FREE | VEGAN | VEGETARIAN

YIELDS 1 SERVING

Ingredients

1 small apple, diced (about 1 cup)
1 tsp cinnamon
1/8 tsp nutmeg
1 pinch cardamom, optional
1/3 cup rolled oats
1 cup non-dairy milk

Directions

1. Add the apples to a small saucepan over medium heat with a lid so the heat creates steam. Let cook for 2 minutes, stirring occasionally.
2. Add the cinnamon, nutmeg, and optional cardamom. Stir together and cook for 1 minute.
3. Add in the oats and non-dairy milk. Cook for 5 minutes, stirring occasionally.
4. Remove from heat and serve immediately.

KCALS 313 | CARBOHYDRATE 68 G | PROTEIN 6 G | FAT 5 G | SATURATED FAT 1 G
SODIUM 84 MG | POTASSIUM 300 MG | FIBER 11 G | CALCIUM 350 MG
PHOSPHORUS 280 MG | IRON 1 MG

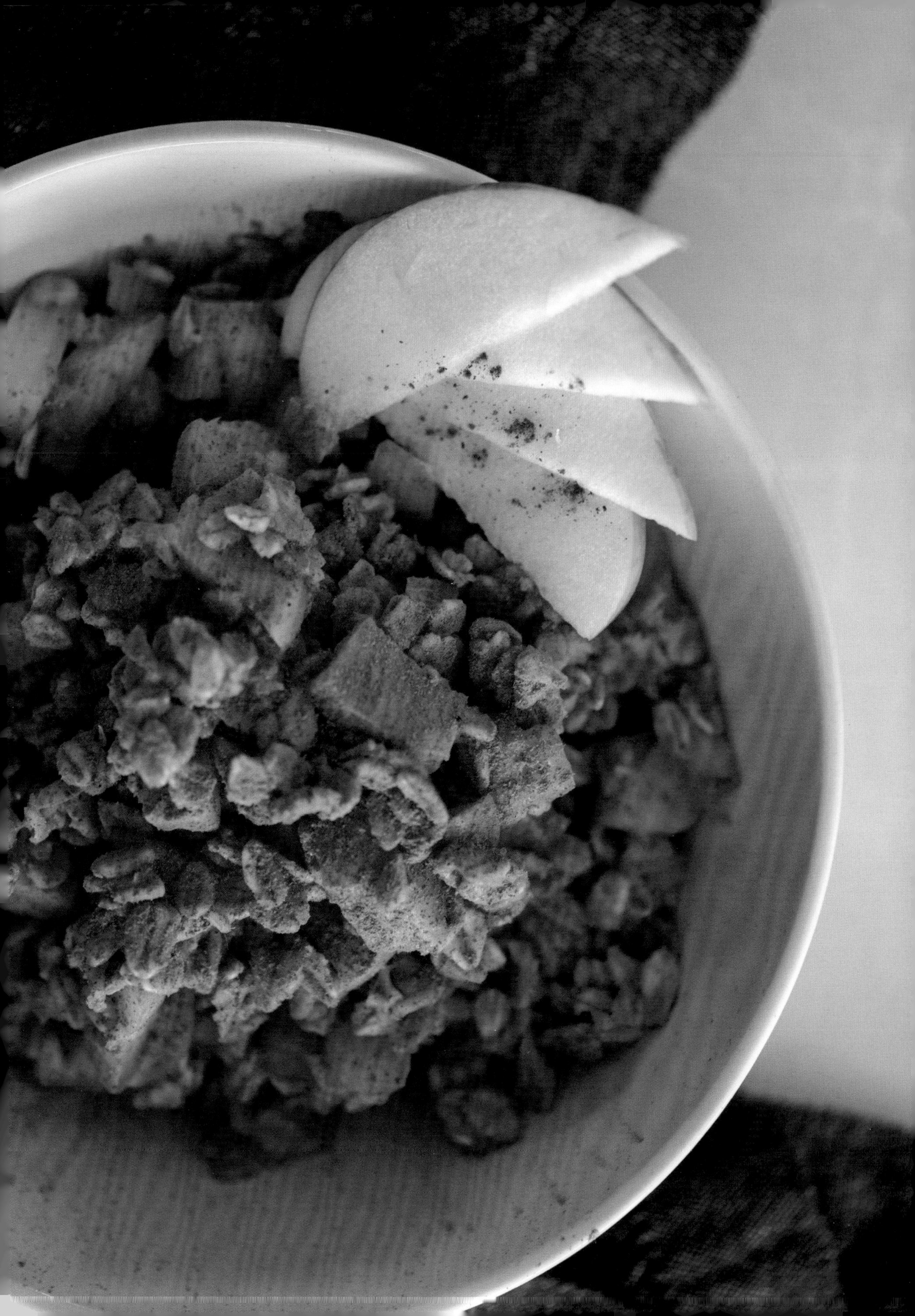

Berry + Granola Parfait

DAIRY-FREE | GLUTEN-FREE | VEGAN | VEGETARIAN

YIELDS 1 SERVING

Ingredients

½ cup homemade granola (page 117)

½ cup fresh berries

1 cup non-dairy milk

Directions

1. Add your granola and berries to a cereal bowl and top with desired non-dairy milk.

KCALS 257 | CARBOHYDRATE 44 G | PROTEIN 4 G | FAT 8 G | SATURATED FAT 3 G
SODIUM 152 MG | POTASSIUM 230 MG | FIBER 11 G | CALCIUM 350 MG
PHOSPHORUS 280 MG | IRON 1 MG

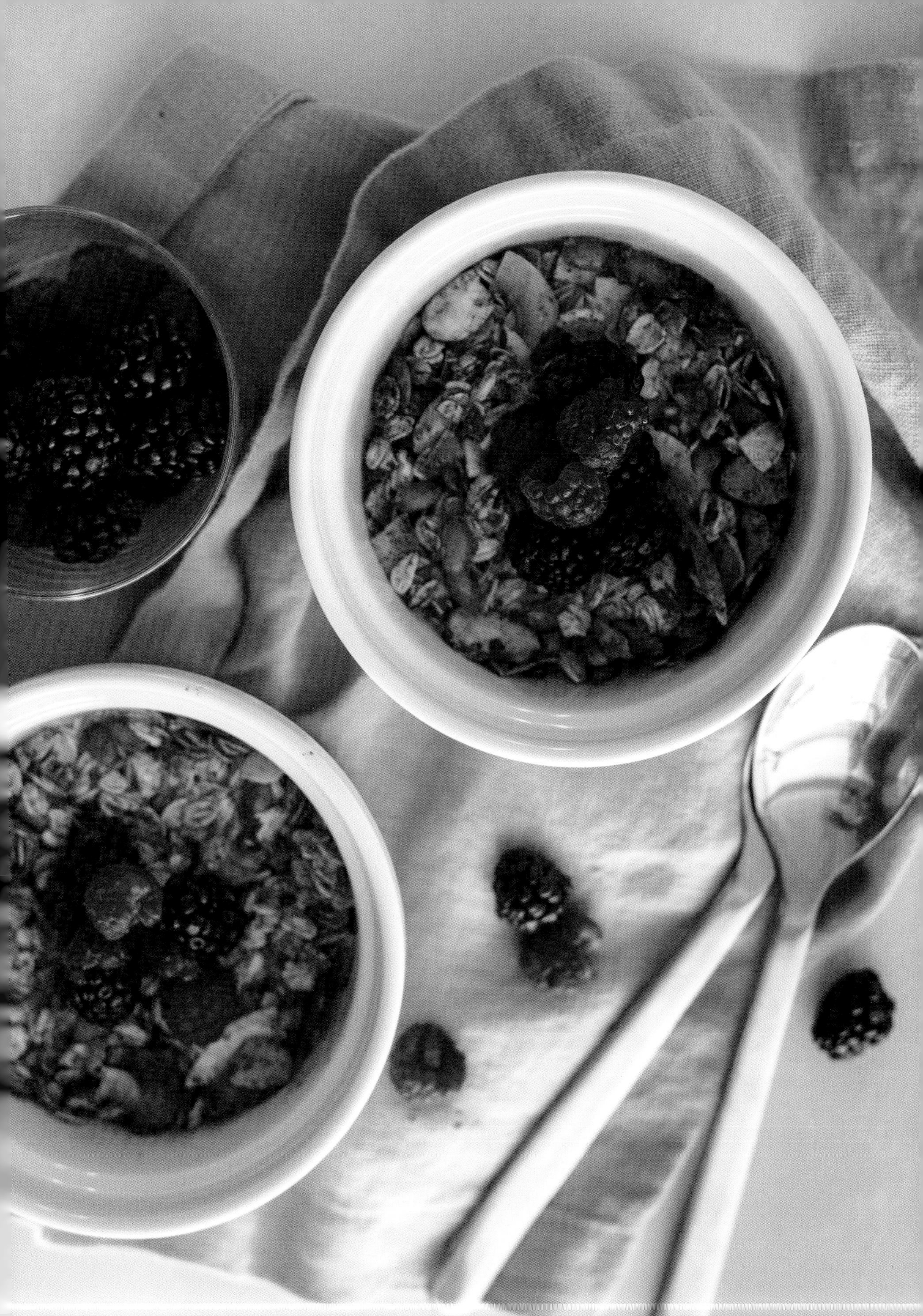

Blueberry Waffles

DAIRY-FREE | GLUTEN-FREE | VEGAN | VEGETARIAN

YIELDS 4-6 SERVINGS DEPENDING ON SIZE OF YOUR WAFFLE IRON. YOU MAY FREEZE THESE AND REHEAT IN THE TOASTER.

Ingredients

1½ cups oat flour
1 tsp baking soda
1 tsp baking powder
1 tsp cinnamon
1 cup almond milk
1 Tbsp lemon juice
2 tsp pure maple syrup
2 tsp vanilla extract
2 Tbsp ground flaxseed +
¼ cup water
¾ cup fresh blueberries

Directions

1. While your waffle iron is heating up, combine your ground flaxseed and water in a small bowl. Stir and set aside.
2. Combine the remaining ingredients in a large mixing bowl and whisk until well combined.
3. Add in your flax and water mixture.
4. Spray your waffle iron with a nonstick spray of your choice.
5. Take about ½–¾ cup of the batter, and pour into your waffle iron.
6. Once cooked, remove from your waffle iron and repeat until your batter is gone.
7. Serve immediately with fresh berries and maple syrup or freeze for a later date.
8. If frozen, simply cook them once more in a toaster before serving.

KCALS 204 | CARBOHYDRATE 36 G | PROTEIN 5 G | FAT 4 G | SATURATED FAT 1 G
SODIUM 316 MG | POTASSIUM 239 MG | FIBER 3 G | CALCIUM 134 MG
PHOSPHORUS 170 MG | IRON 2 MG

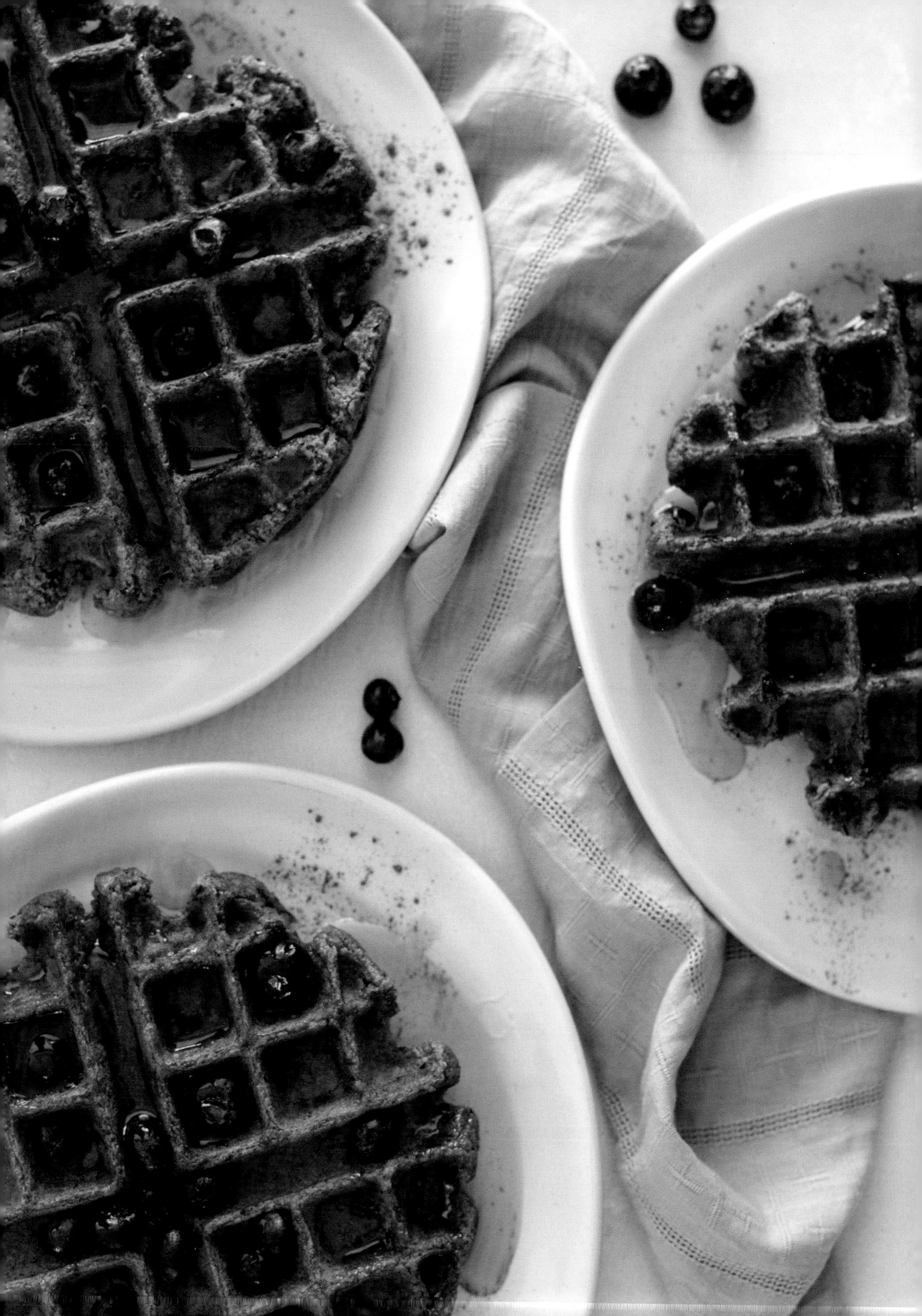

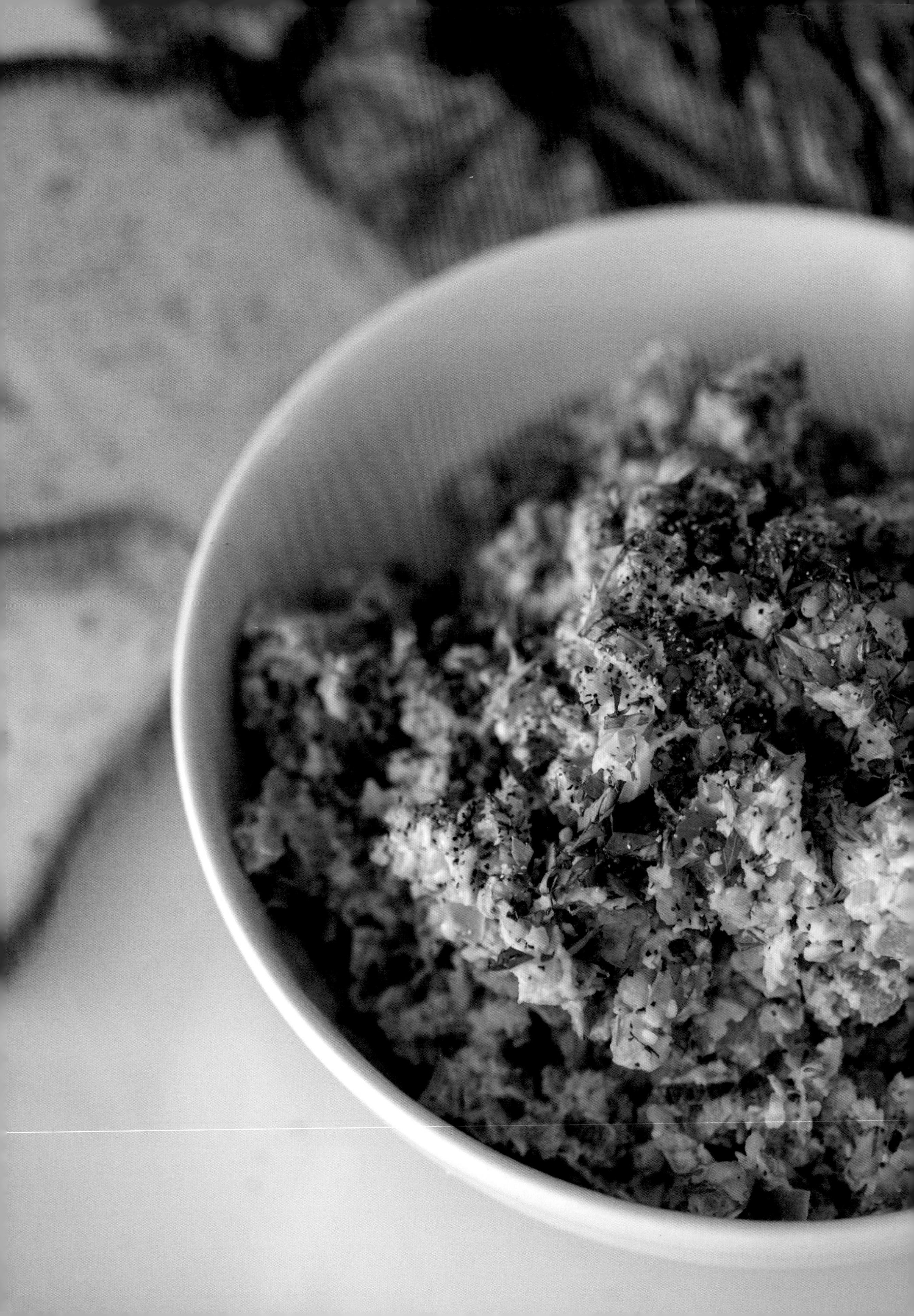

LUNCH

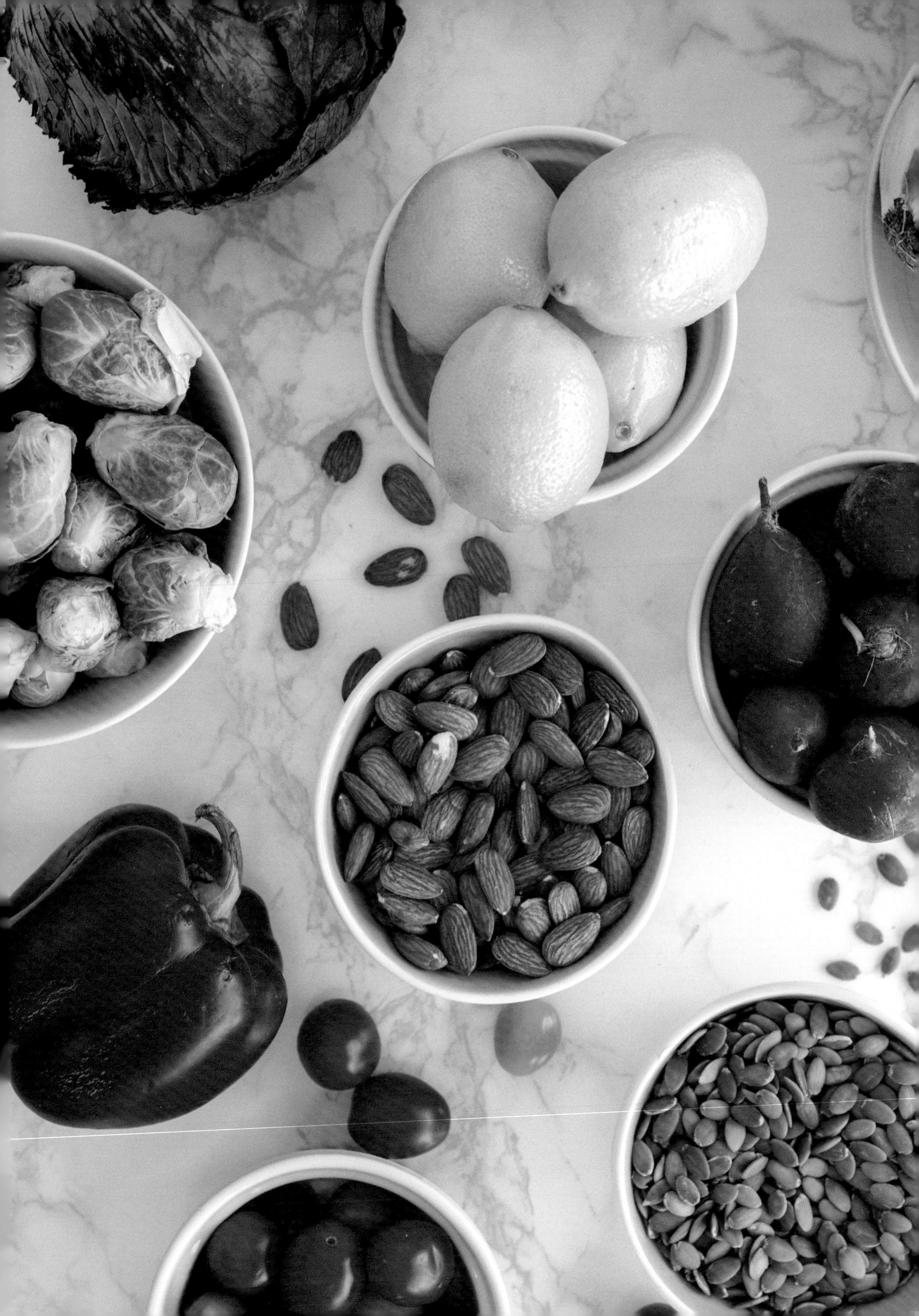

BUILD YOUR OWN SALAD

LEAFY GREENS

ARUGULA
KALE
ROMAINE
BUTTER LETTUCE
SPINACH
SPROUTS

VEGGIES

TOMATOES
BELL PEPPER
CUCUMBER
CABBAGE
RADISH
CARROT
CELERY
ONION
1/4 AVOCADO

DRESSINGS

OLIVE OIL
LEMON JUICE
BALSAMIC VINEGAR
RED WINE VINEGAR
CHAMPAGNE VINEGAR
LOW SODIUM DRESSINGS

BEAN & LEGUMES

1/4 CUP CHICKPEAS
1/4 CUP BLACK BEANS
1/4 CUP KIDNEY BEANS
1/4 CUP LENTILS
1/4 CUP TOFU
1/4 CUP TEMPEH

NUTS & SEEDS

ALMONDS
PECANS
WALNUTS
PISTACHIOS
MACADAMIA NUTS
PUMPKIN SEEDS
SUNFLOWER SEEDS

Chopped Salad with Basil Ranch Dressing

DAIRY-FREE | GLUTEN-FREE | VEGAN | VEGETARIAN

YIELDS 6 SERVINGS

Creamy Basil Ranch Dressing Ingredients

¾ cup raw cashews
¾ cup filtered water
1 Tbsp apple cider vinegar
2 cloves garlic, smashed and peeled
1 tsp onion powder
½ tsp sea salt
1 tsp ground black pepper
½ cup fresh basil, finely chopped
¼ cup fresh chives, finely chopped

Chopped Salad Ingredients

1 can of chickpeas, drained and rinsed, tossed with 1Tbsp olive oil, 1 tsp smoked paprika, 1 tsp cumin, ¼ tsp salt, and ½ tsp pepper, and roasted until crispy
1 medium-large zucchini, diced
1 large head romaine, washed and thoroughly chopped
1 cup baby kale or spring mix
2 stalks celery, diced
2 medium carrots, peeled, quartered lengthwise and thinly sliced
1 cup diced cherry tomatoes
¼ cup raw shelled sunflower seeds, to taste
Freshly ground black pepper, to taste

Directions

1. Preheat oven to 425°F.
2. Rinse and drain chickpeas, if you haven't already. Toss chickpeas with 1 Tbsp olive oil, 1 tsp smoked paprika, 1 tsp cumin, ¼ tsp salt, and ½ tsp pepper.
3. Roast chickpeas on a baking sheet in the oven for 15–20 minutes, or until crispy.
4. Blend all ingredients for the dressing in a blender EXCEPT the basil and chives. Once creamy, stir in the basil and chives and set the dressing aside or store in fridge.
5. Chop all other salad ingredients and combine in a large bowl.

KCALS 246 | CARBOHYDRATE 26 G | PROTEIN 10 G | FAT 13 G | SATURATED FAT 2 G
SODIUM 61 MG | POTASSIUM 759 MG | FIBER 9 G | CALCIUM 107 MG
PHOSPHORUS 332 MG | IRON 3 MG

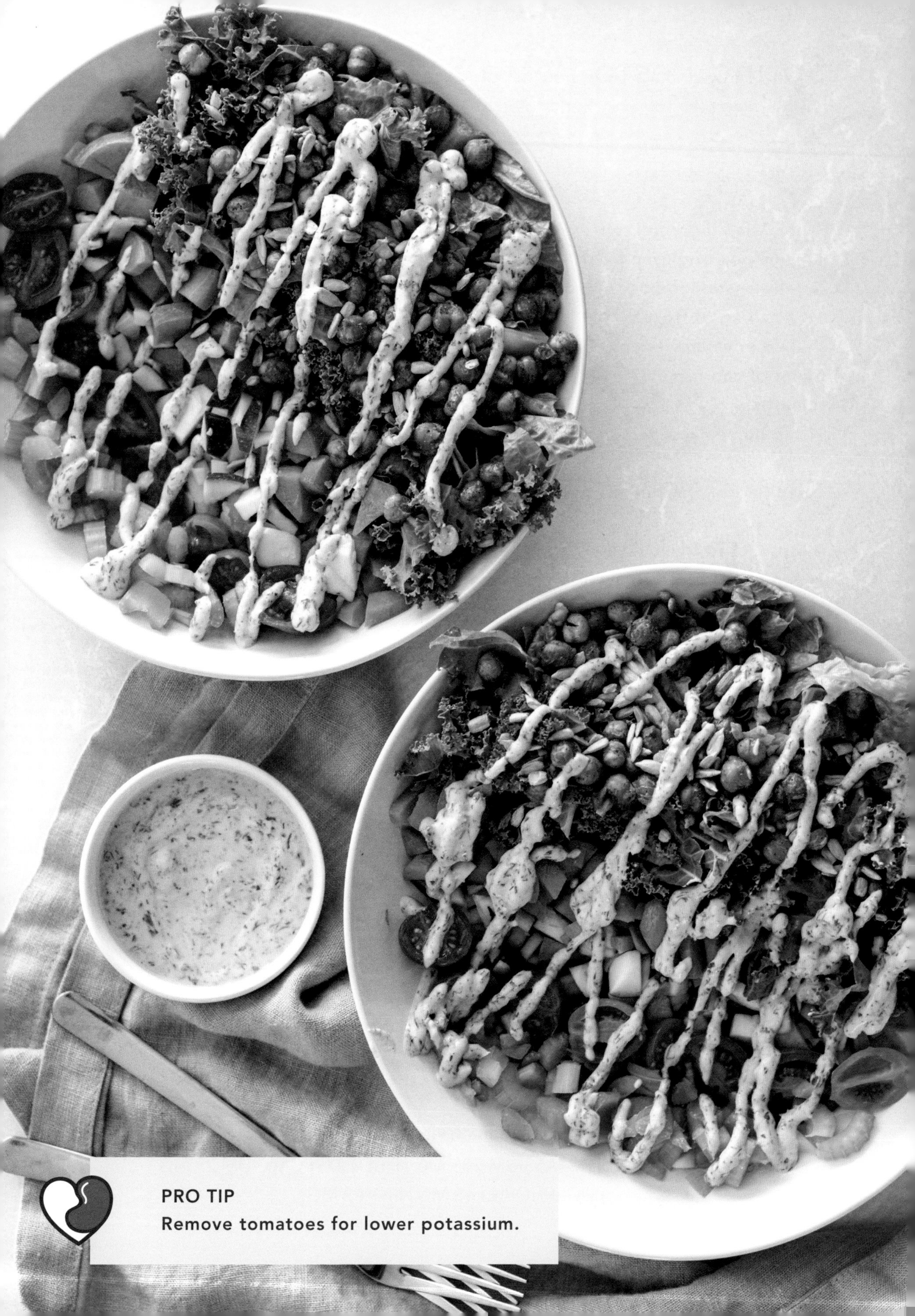

PRO TIP
Remove tomatoes for lower potassium.

Spring Pesto Pasta Salad

DAIRY-FREE | GLUTEN-FREE | VEGAN | VEGETARIAN

YIELDS 8 SERVINGS

Pasta Salad Ingredients

1 12-oz box of gluten-free farfalle pasta noodles
1 12-oz bag of frozen shelled edamame beans
1 pint of cherry tomatoes
¾ cup homemade pesto

Pesto Sauce Ingredients

(Yields 3/4 cup)

1 cup packed fresh basil
¾ cup packed fresh parsley
¼ cup raw pine nuts or pumpkin seeds
2 garlic cloves
¼ cup extra virgin olive oil
¼ cup lemon juice
½ tsp salt

Directions

1. Cook noodles according to package directions.
2. While noodles cook, make pesto sauce, dice tomatoes, and thaw edamame beans.
3. Once everything is ready, combine all ingredients in a large bowl and toss until the pesto is thoroughly incorporated.
4. Serve immediately or store in an airtight container in the refrigerator for up to 7 days.

Pesto Sauce Directions

1. Place all ingredients in a food processor or blender and pulse or blend until smooth and well combined.

KCALS 318 | CARBOHYDRATE 45 G | PROTEIN 7 G | FAT 14 G | SATURATED FAT 2 G
SODIUM 186 MG | POTASSIUM 205 MG | FIBER 2 G | CALCIUM 23 MG
PHOSPHORUS 48 MG | IRON 2 MG

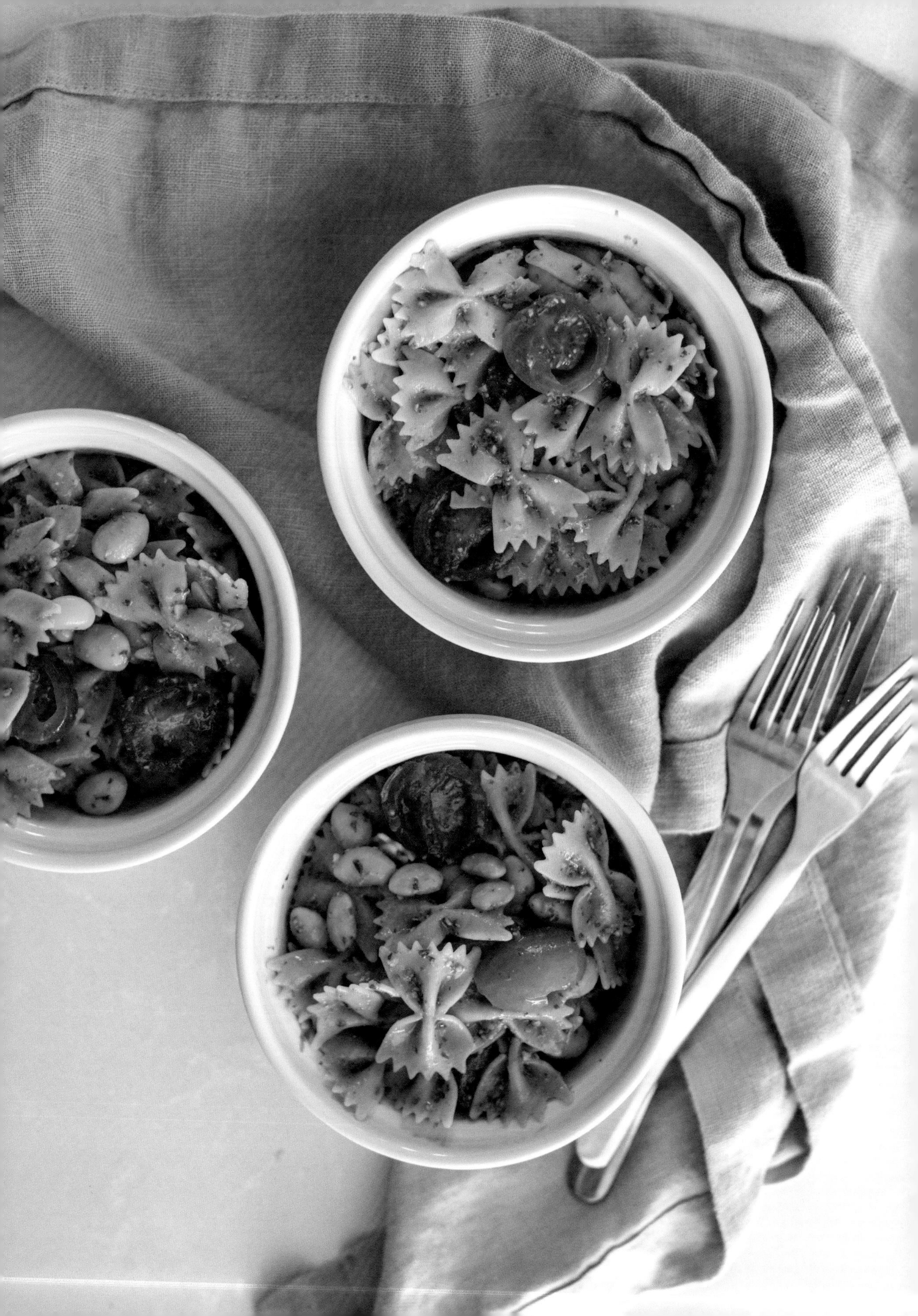

Chickpea Salad

DAIRY-FREE | GLUTEN-FREE | NUT-FREE | VEGAN | VEGETARIAN

YIELDS 6 SERVINGS

Ingredients

2 cans of no salt added chickpeas, rinsed and drained
1 green bell pepper, diced
1 bunch green onions, diced
3 celery stalks, diced
2 Tbsp fresh dill, chopped
1/2 cup raw and unsalted sunflower seeds
1/4 cup hemp seeds
1/3 cup tahini
1 Tbsp fresh lemon juice
1 Tbsp dijon mustard
Salt and pepper to taste

Directions

1. Once you have drained and rinsed your chickpeas, pour them into a large mixing bowl. Use a fork or potato masher to break them down and slightly mash them.
2. Add in diced vegetables (bell pepper, green onion, celery, and dill) and stir well.
3. Add in tahini, lemon juice, mustard, hemp seeds, and sunflower seeds. Stir until well combined.
4. Salt and pepper to taste.
5. Store in an airtight container for up to 7 days.
6. Serve with lettuce wraps or crackers, or as a sandwich. (We recommend using gluten free crackers or bread where possible.)

KCALS 318 | CARBOHYDRATE 27 G | PROTEIN 14 G | FAT 19 G | SATURATED FAT 2 G
SODIUM 60 MG | POTASSIUM 493 MG | FIBER 9 G | CALCIUM 92 MG
PHOSPHORUS 406 MG | IRON 3 MG

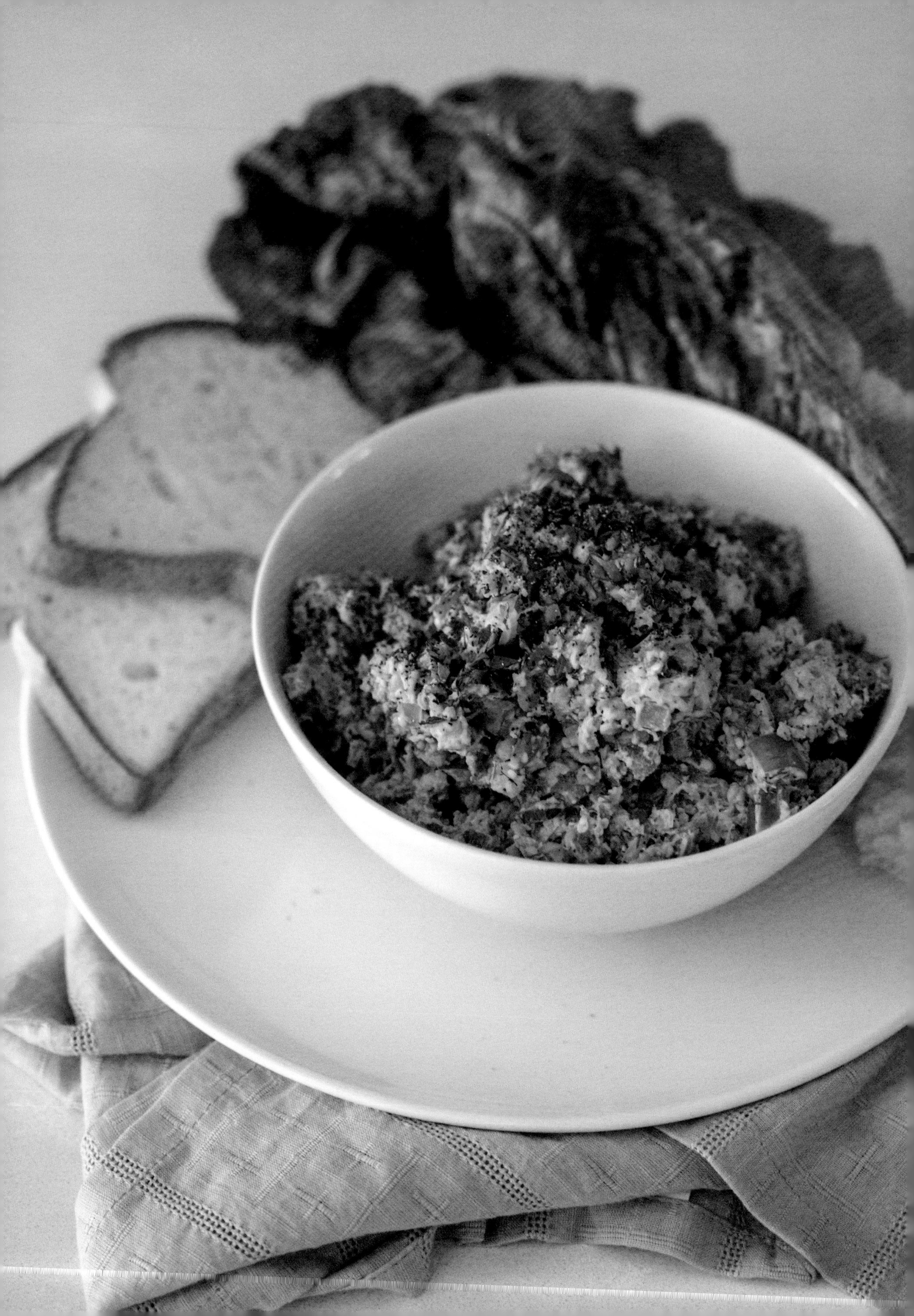

5-Minute Veggie Sandwich

DAIRY-FREE | GLUTEN-FREE | NUT-FREE | VEGAN | VEGETARIAN

YIELDS 1 SERVING

Ingredients

2 pieces of gluten free bread
¼ cup hummus
½ avocado
½ roma tomato
¼ bell pepper
½ cup spinach
¼ cup broccoli sprouts

Directions

1. Toast your sandwich bread until warm and lightly crispy.
2. Spread hummus onto both pieces of bread.
3. Top with your avocado, tomato, bell pepper, lettuce, sprouts, and any other desired ingredients.
4. Put it together as a sandwich and enjoy!

YOU'VE GOT OPTIONS!

- Need lower potassium? Simply remove the avocado.
- Don't like spinach? Try arugula!
- Pro tip: Add a dollop of our homemade pesto from page 85!

KCALS 366 | CARBOHYDRATE 43 G | PROTEIN 6 G | FAT 20 G | SATURATED FAT 2 G
SODIUM 244 MG | POTASSIUM 688 MG | FIBER 10 G | CALCIUM 103 MG
PHOSPHORUS 80 MG | IRON 1 MG

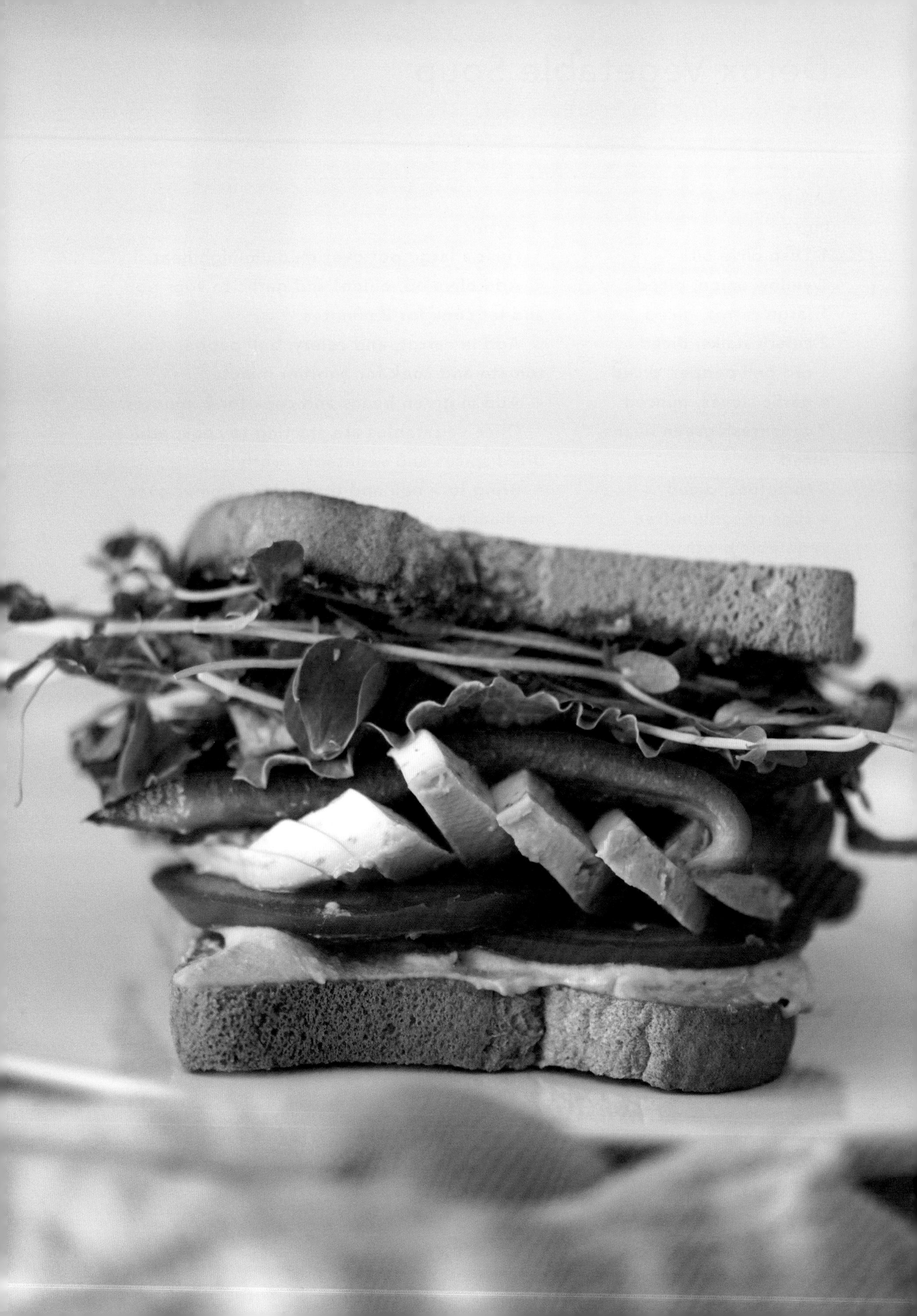

Detox Vegetable Soup

DAIRY-FREE | GLUTEN-FREE | VEGAN | NUT-FREE | VEGETARIAN

YIELDS 8 SERVINGS

Ingredients

1 Tbsp olive oil
1 yellow onion, diced
1 large carrot, diced
2 celery stalks, diced
1 red bell pepper, diced
4 garlic cloves, minced
2 cups fresh green beans, diced
3 tomatoes, diced
4 cups of sodium-free vegetable broth
2 tsp dried oregano
1 tsp dried basil
1 tsp dried thyme
1 tsp sea salt
½ tsp black pepper
4 cups kale
2 Tbsp fresh parsley

Directions

1. Heat a large pot over medium-high heat.
2. Add olive oil, onion, and garlic to your pot and let cook for 2 minutes.
3. Add in carrot, and celery, bell pepper, and tomato and cook for another minute.
4. Add in green beans and cook for 2 minutes.
5. Once vegetables are starting to cook, add dried spices and vegetable broth.
6. Bring to a boil and then let it summer over medium heat for about 20–25 minutes.
7. Add in kale at the very end, and only cook for about 4–5 minutes.
8. When you're ready to serve, top each bowl with fresh parsley and enjoy!
9. Store in the refrigerator for up to a week or freeze for a later date.

KCALS 73 | CARBOHYDRATE 12 G | PROTEIN 2 G | FAT 3 G | SATURATED FAT 0 G
SODIUM 114 MG | POTASSIUM 346 MG | FIBER 3 G | CALCIUM 52 MG
PHOSPHORUS 44 MG | IRON 1 MG

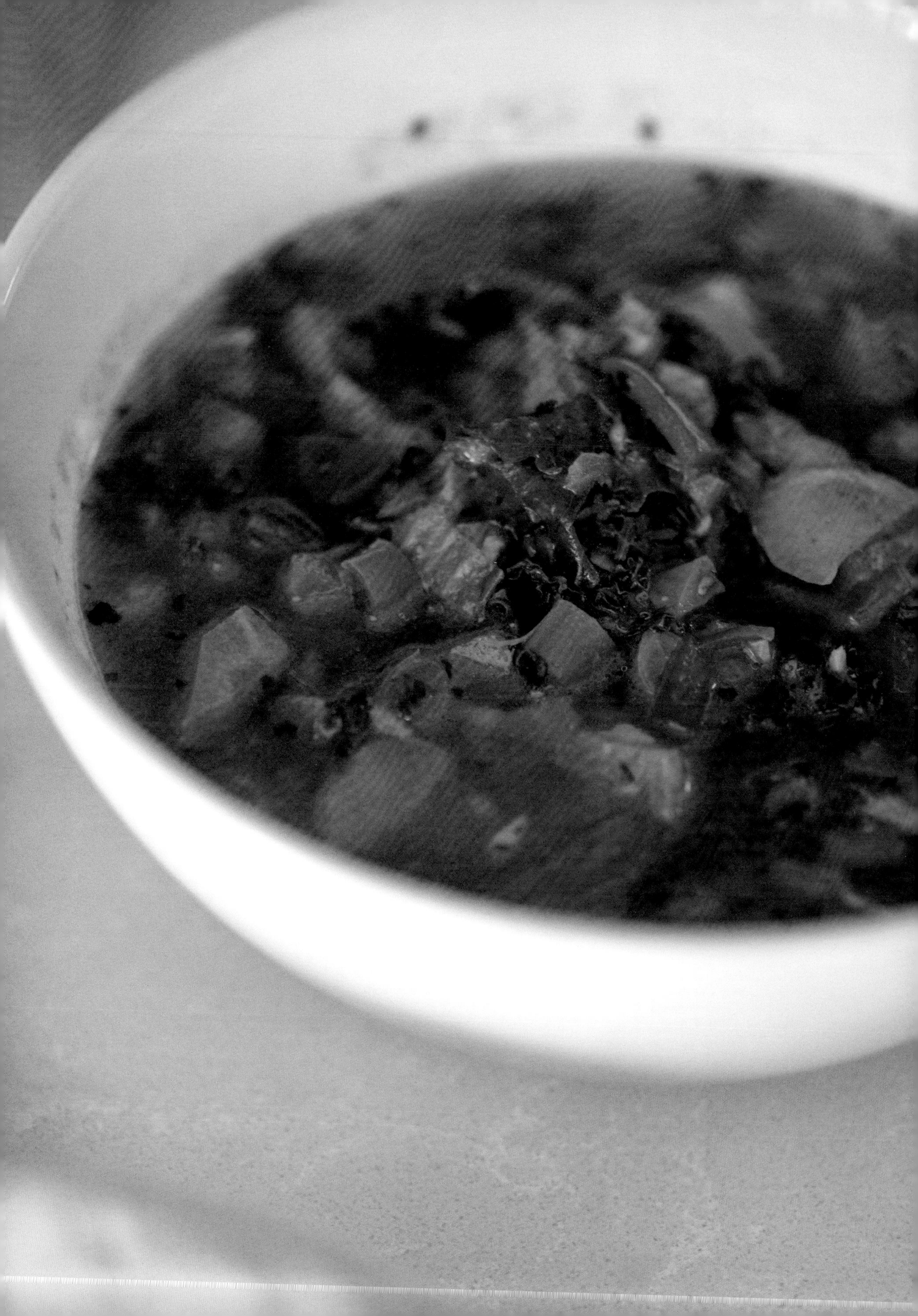

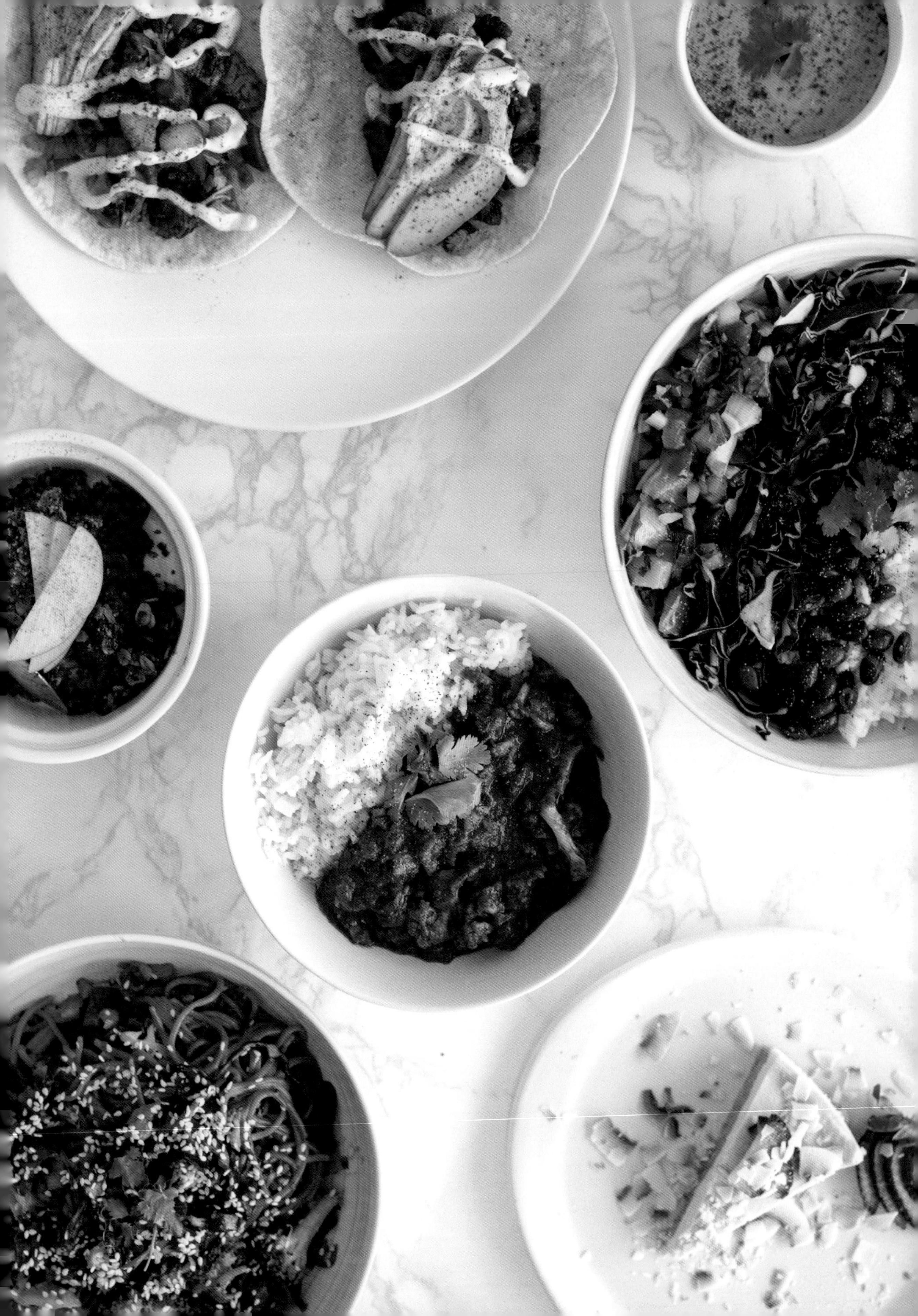

DINNER

Almond Alfredo Pasta with Roasted Broccolini

DAIRY-FREE | GLUTEN-FREE | VEGAN | VEGETARIAN

YIELDS 4 SERVINGS

Misc. Ingredients

1 box of gluten-free pasta
1 bunch of broccolini
1 Tbsp garlic, minced
2 Tbsp olive oil
½ tsp black pepper

Sauce Ingredients

½ cup almonds
½ cup cashews
1¼ cups water
¼ cup nutritional yeast
1 Tbsp garlic
1 Tbsp dried parsley
1 lemon, juiced
½ tsp salt
1 tsp black pepper

Directions

1. Preheat oven to 375°F.
2. Bring a pot of water to boil.
3. Place broccolini on a baking sheet and toss with minced garlic, olive oil, and pepper. Bake for 15–18 minutes, or until cooked through and slightly crispy.
4. While water heats up, blend all sauce ingredients on high until smooth and creamy. Once done, set aside.
5. Once water is boiling, cook pasta according to box directions. When they are cooked and you are ready to strain them, be sure to keep 1–2 cups of pasta water just in case you wish to thin out your sauce.
6. Remove broccolini from oven and set aside.
7. Pour alfredo sauce onto noodles and stir until well combined. If desired, pour the remaining pasta water in, ¼ cup at a time until you reach your desired creaminess.
8. Serve pasta immediately and top with roasted broccolini.
9. Leftover sauce will last for up to 7 days when stored in an airtight container in the refrigerator.

KCALS 585 | CARBOHYDRATE 84 G | PROTEIN 17 G | FAT 25 G | SATURATED FAT 3 G
SODIUM 330 MG | POTASSIUM 483 MG | FIBER 9 G | CALCIUM 112 MG
PHOSPHORUS 265 MG | IRON 3 MG

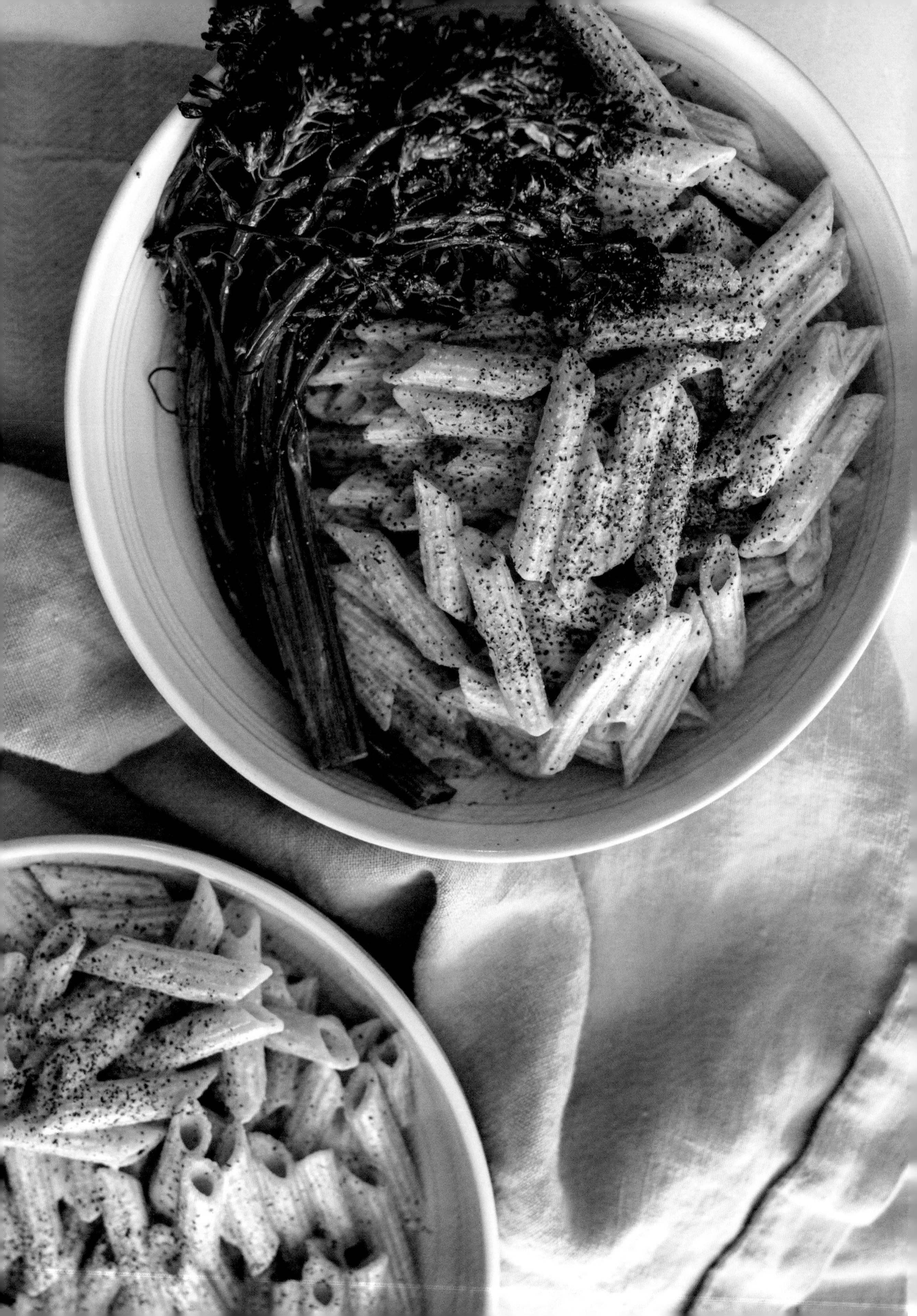

Black Bean & Sweet Potato Burgers

DAIRY-FREE | GLUTEN-FREE | VEGAN | NUT-FREE | VEGETARIAN

YIELDS 6 BURGER PATTIES

Ingredients

1 large sweet potato
½ cup raw quinoa
1, 15-oz can of no salt added black beans
½ cup finely diced red onion
1/3 cup chopped fresh cilantro
3 garlic cloves
2 tsp smoked paprika
2 tsp ground cumin
½ tsp salt
¾ cup quick-cooking oats

Directions

1. Preheat oven to 400°F.
2. If you haven't already, dice sweet potato into small squares. Place diced sweet potato on a parchment paper-lined baking sheet and bake in the oven for 30 minutes, or until the sweet potatoes are soft and you can stick a fork through them.
3. While the potatoes are cooking, cook the quinoa. Place ½ cup of raw quinoa in a pot with 1 cup of water. Bring to a boil and then let simmer for about 10 minutes, or until all of the water is absorbed.
4. Chop onion and cilantro, mince garlic, and drain and rinse black beans.
5. In the base of your food processor, add onion, cilantro, garlic, cumin, smoked paprika, and salt.
6. Once quinoa and sweet potatoes are done cooking, add them to the onion mix in the food processor. The only ingredient you do not want in the food processor yet are the black beans.
7. Blend or process the mix until it is well combined and sticks together like a dough. It won't take long, and it's best to not over-blend. You should still see chunks of onion and whole pieces of quinoa.

Directions continued →

KCALS 192 | CARBOHYDRATE 7 G | PROTEIN 7 G | FAT 1 G | SATURATED FAT 1 G
SODIUM 230 MG | POTASSIUM 592 MG | FIBER 7 G | CALCIUM 63 MG
PHOSPHORUS 117 MG | IRON 3 MG

8. Add in black beans and process for a few more moments. You want your beans to be broken down and well-combined into the rest of the mix, but you don't want them to be completely mushy.
9. Once you have a dough that sticks together, transfer it to a regular mixing bowl.
10. Add in your quick oats and stir until well combined. The oats will help dry it out and make it stick together.
11. When you're ready to mold your burgers, gently roll about ½ cup of dough into a ball and then flatten into the shape of a burger.
12. Cook burgers on the stovetop for about 2 minutes on each side, or grill them like you would a traditional burger.
13. Serve with all of your favorite burger toppings or enjoy your black bean patty on a salad or wrap of your choice.

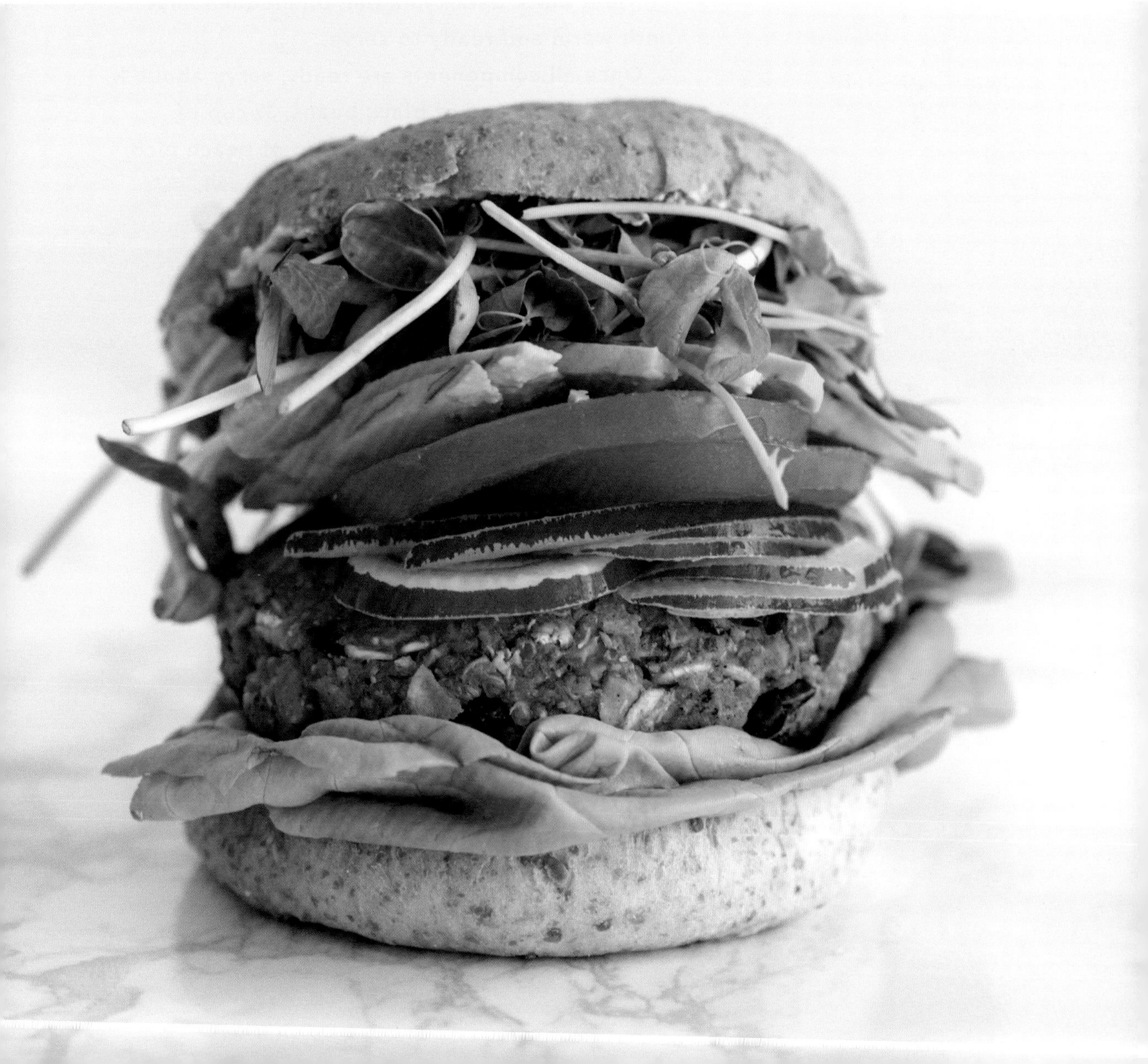

Burrito Bowl

DAIRY-FREE | GLUTEN-FREE | VEGAN | NUT-FREE | VEGETARIAN

YIELDS 6 SERVINGS

Ingredients

2 cups dry rice
2, 15-oz cans of no salt added black beans
1 batch peach pico (page 125)
2 cups shredded purple cabbage
Cilantro for topping

Directions

1. In a pot on the stove, cook rice according to package directions. Typically, you will cook 2 cups of rice with 4 cups of water over medium heat for about 20 minutes, or until all of the water is absorbed. When your rice is done cooking, set it to the side.
2. While rice is cooking, make peach pico (page 125) and set to the side once done.
3. Heat black beans in a pan on medium heat until warm and ready to serve.
4. Once all components are ready, serve about 1 cup of rice, ½ cup of black beans, ½ cup of shredded purple cabbage, ½ cup of peach pico, and a few leaves of cilantro in each bowl.

PRO TIP
Drizzle with our homemade cashew queso recipe from page 123.

KCALS 318 | CARBOHYDRATE 68 G | PROTEIN 9 G | FAT 2 G | SATURATED FAT 2 G
SODIUM 17 MG | POTASSIUM 553 MG | FIBER 6 G | CALCIUM 64 MG
PHOSPHORUS 289 MG | IRON 5 MG

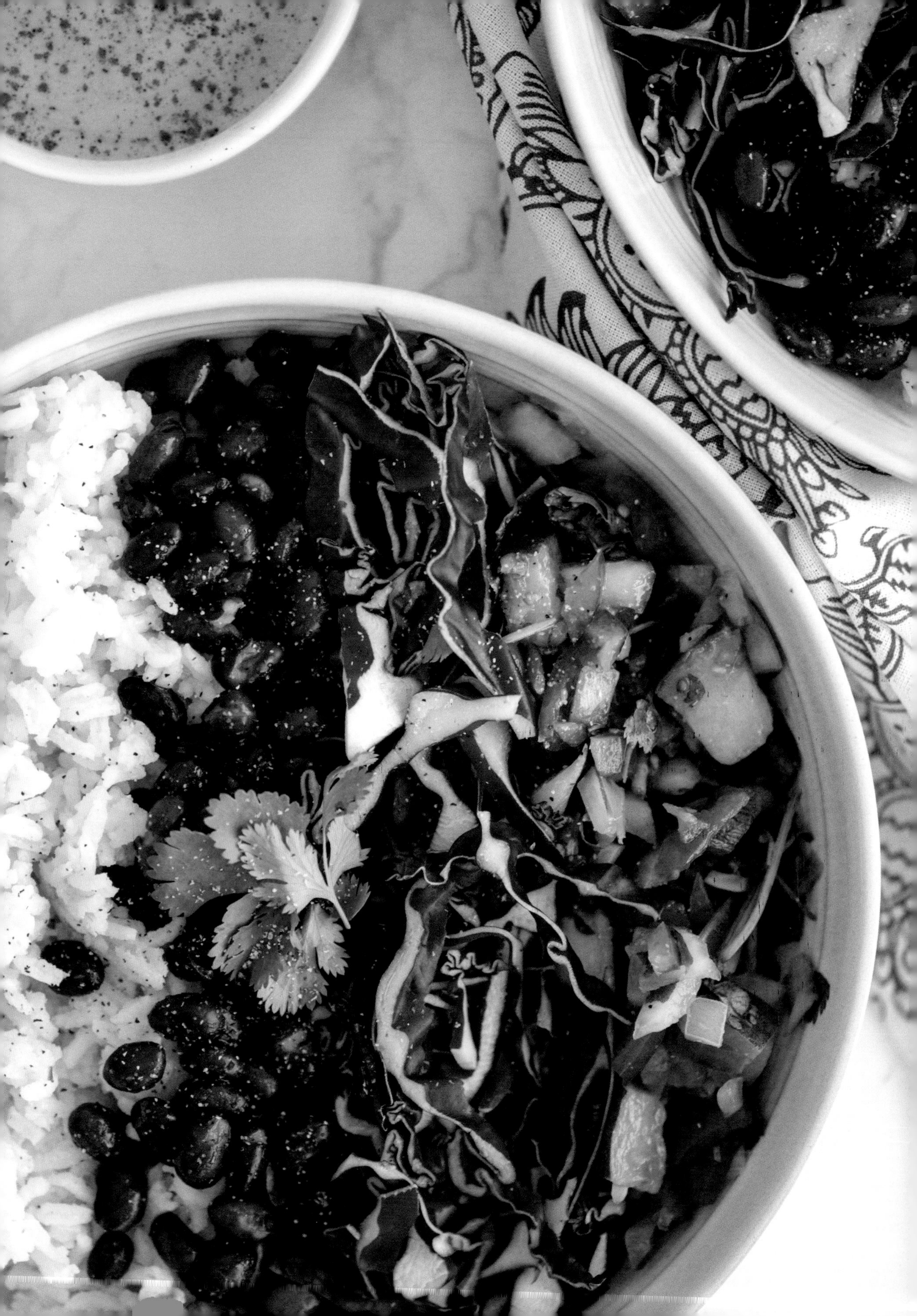

Pesto Buddha Bowl

DAIRY-FREE | GLUTEN-FREE | VEGAN | VEGETARIAN

YIELDS 6 SERVINGS

Ingredients

2 cups of dry rice
1 head of cauliflower
3–4 cups of Brussels sprouts
1 batch pesto sauce (page 85)
1 Tbsp olive oil
1/2 tsp salt
1/2 tsp black pepper

Directions

1. Preheat oven to 375°F.
2. Dice cauliflower and Brussels sprouts and place in a large bowl.
3. Toss cauliflower and Brussels sprout mix with 1 Tbsp olive oil, ½ tsp salt, and ½ tsp black pepper. Once well combined, evenly place on a baking sheet and bake for 30–35 minutes, or until they are cooked through and have a slight crisp on the outside.
4. While vegetables are cooking, cook your rice according to package directions in a pot on the stove. Typically, you will cook 2 cups of rice with 4 cups of water over medium heat for about 20 minutes, or until all of the water is absorbed. When rice is done cooking, set it to the side.
5. While rice is cooking, make pesto sauce (page 85) and set to the side once done.
6. Once all components are ready, serve about 1 cup of rice with 1½ cups of the Brussels sprout and cauliflower mix per person. Top with your desired amount of pesto and enjoy!

CHECK OUT OUR PESTO SAUCE ON PAGE 85.

KCALS 422 | CARBOHYDRATE 59 G | PROTEIN 9 G | FAT 18 G | SATURATED FAT 3 G
SODIUM 144 MG | POTASSIUM 727 MG | FIBER 10 G | CALCIUM 81 MG
PHOSPHORUS 280 MG | IRON 3 MG

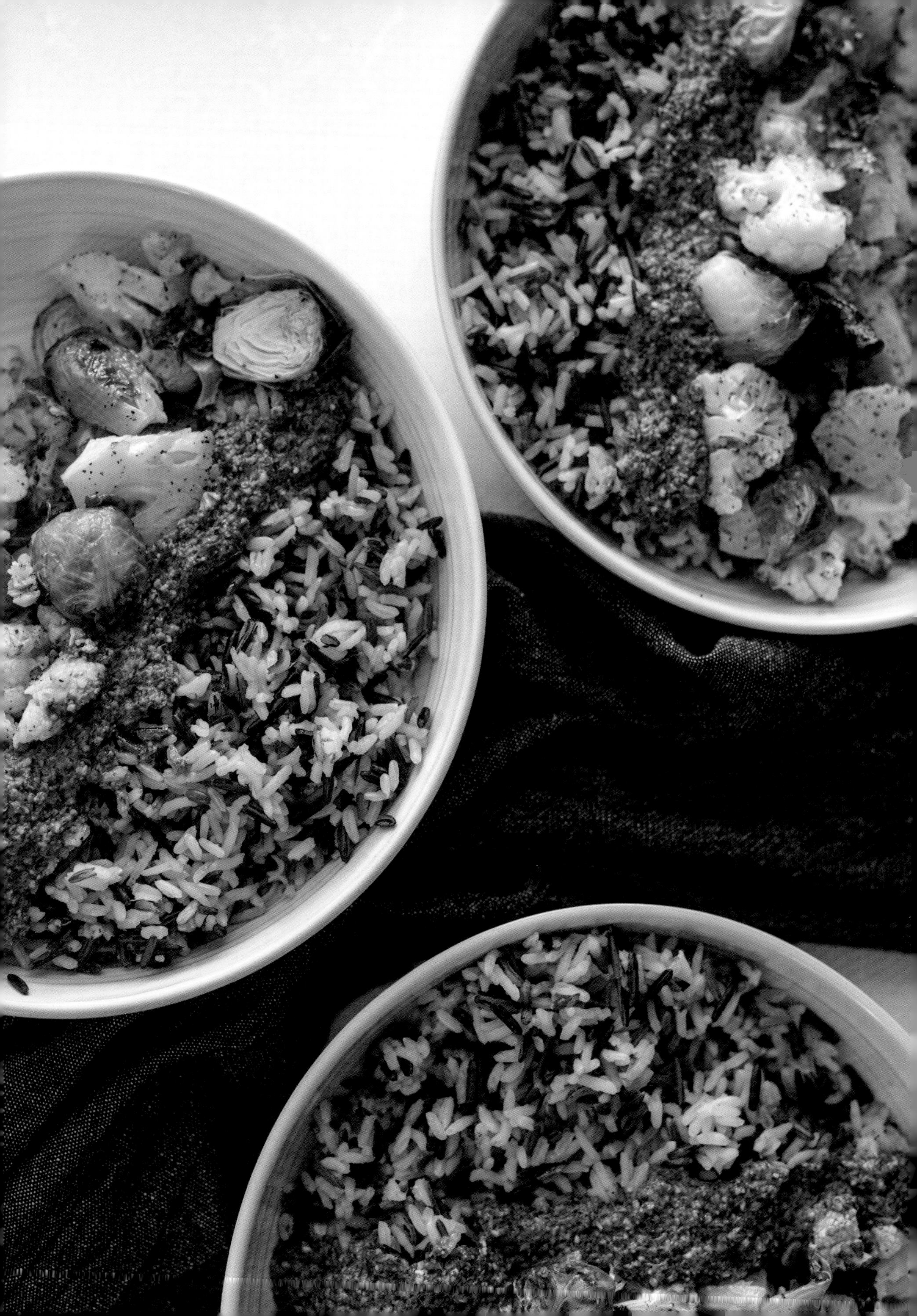

Lentil Sloppy Joes

DAIRY-FREE | GLUTEN-FREE | VEGAN | VEGETARIAN

YIELDS 6 SERVINGS

Ingredients

1½ cups dry green lentils
1 yellow onion, diced
3 cloves garlic, minced
½ red bell pepper, diced
1 can no salt added tomato sauce
2 Tbsp Worcestershire sauce
3 Tbsp coconut sugar
1 Tbsp chili powder
½ Tbsp cumin
½ Tbsp smoked paprika
½ tsp black pepper
6 gluten free hamburger buns or 12 slider buns of choice

Directions

You can make these one of two ways. I like to cook the lentils in a rice cooker or Instant Pot and then add them to a sauté pan with all of the other ingredients. Instead, you may cook the lentils in a sauté pan and add in all of your other ingredients simultaneously. Both options work great!

1. While your lentils are cooking, sauté all of your ingredients in a medium-large sized sauté pan. Once the onions are cooked and your lentils are done, stir in your lentils until the sauce mixture is well combined.
2. Serve immediately on a bun or lettuce wrap of your choosing or store in the refrigerator for up to 1 week.

HEALTH REMINDERS!

- If you are strictly vegan, be sure to use a vegan Worcestershire sauce.
- Lettuce wraps make a great bun replacement!

KCALS 271 | CARBOHYDRATE 54 G | PROTEIN 11 G | FAT 3 G | SATURATED FAT 1 G
SODIUM 273 MG | POTASSIUM 541 MG | FIBER 6 G | CALCIUM 102 MG
PHOSPHORUS 170 MG | IRON 5 MG

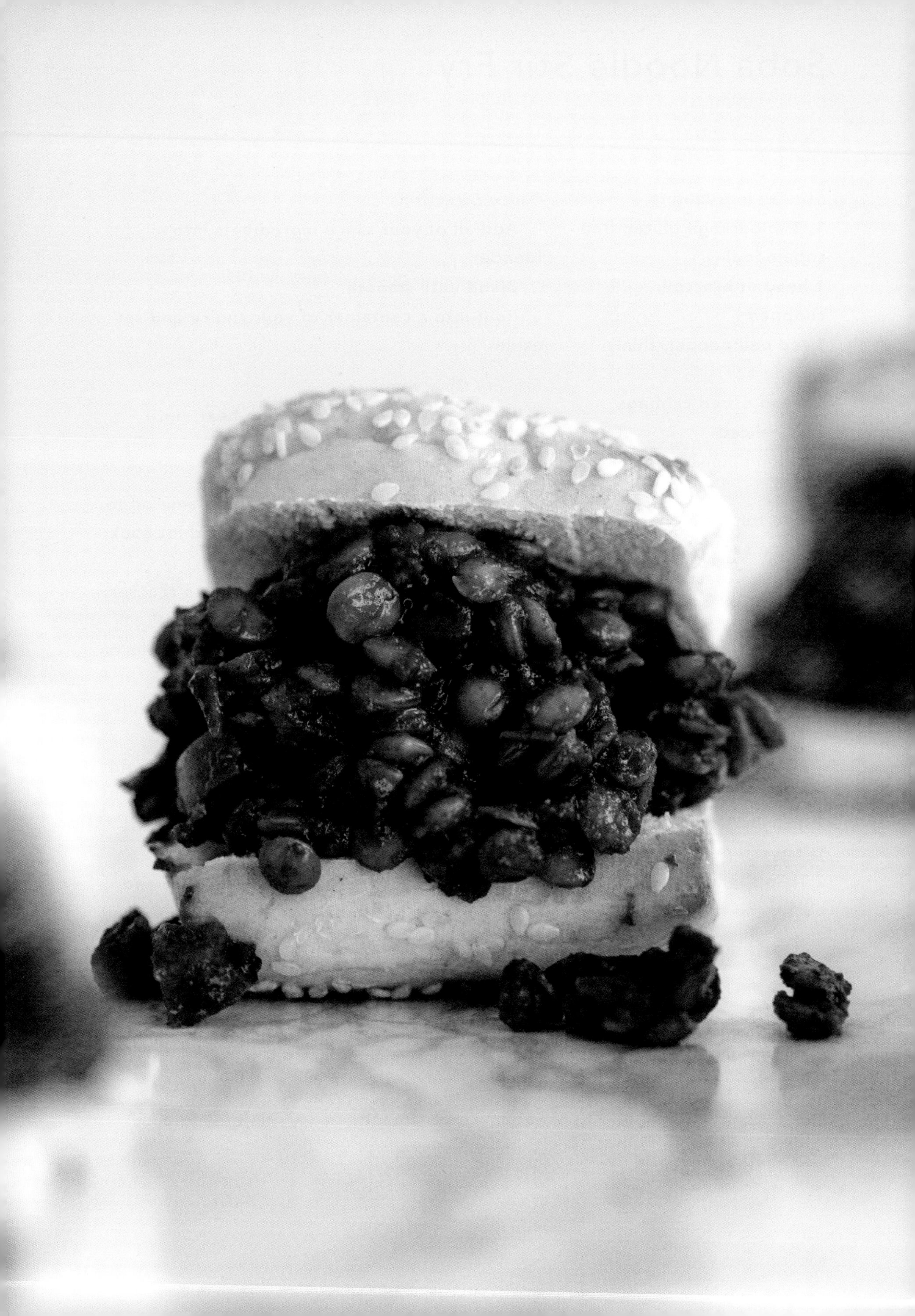

Soba Noodle Stir Fry

DAIRY-FREE | GLUTEN-FREE | VEGAN | NUT-FREE | VEGETARIAN

YIELDS 6 SERVINGS

Stir Fry Ingredients

1, 1 lb package gluten free soba noodles
1 head of broccoli, chopped
1 red bell pepper, thinly sliced
¼ head of red cabbage, thinly sliced
4 green onions, thinly sliced
¼ cup fresh chopped basil
Sesame seeds for garnish
1 Tbsp of toasted sesame oil

Sauce Ingredients

¼ cup coconut aminos
2 Tbsp rice wine vinegar
2 Tbsp pure maple syrup
1 Tbsp toasted sesame oil
2 garlic cloves
1 inch knob fresh ginger
½ tsp red pepper flakes
2 Tbsp sunflower seed butter (no salt & no sugar)

Sauce Directions

1. Add all of your sauce ingredients into a blender.
2. Blend until smooth.
3. Pour into a container of your choice and set aside.

Stir Fry Directions

1. Heat a pot of water over high heat, until boiling.
2. Heat a skillet over medium heat.
3. Add one tablespoon of toasted sesame oil to your skillet. Then add the broccoli and let cook for 3-4 minutes.
4. Add cabbage and red bell pepper to the skillet. Combine well.
5. Once pot of water is boiling, cook noodles on medium heat for 5 minutes.
6. Cook vegetable mixture for 5 minutes, while noodles boil.
7. Once soft, strain noodles and rinse with cold water so they don't overcook.
8. Add noodles to vegetable mixture and toss well.
9. Pour about ½ of sauce onto the stir fry and toss well. Then, add the remaining sauce or wait to do so until serving.
10. For serving, top each serving with fresh basil, green onion, sesame seeds, and more sauce if needed.

HEALTH FACTS
Coconut aminos is a healthier version of soy sauce.

KCALS 279 | CARBOHYDRATE 43 G | PROTEIN 10 G | FAT 9 G | SATURATED FAT 1 G
SODIUM 273 MG | POTASSIUM 568 MG | FIBER 5 G | CALCIUM 73 MG
PHOSPHORUS 110 MG | IRON 2 MG

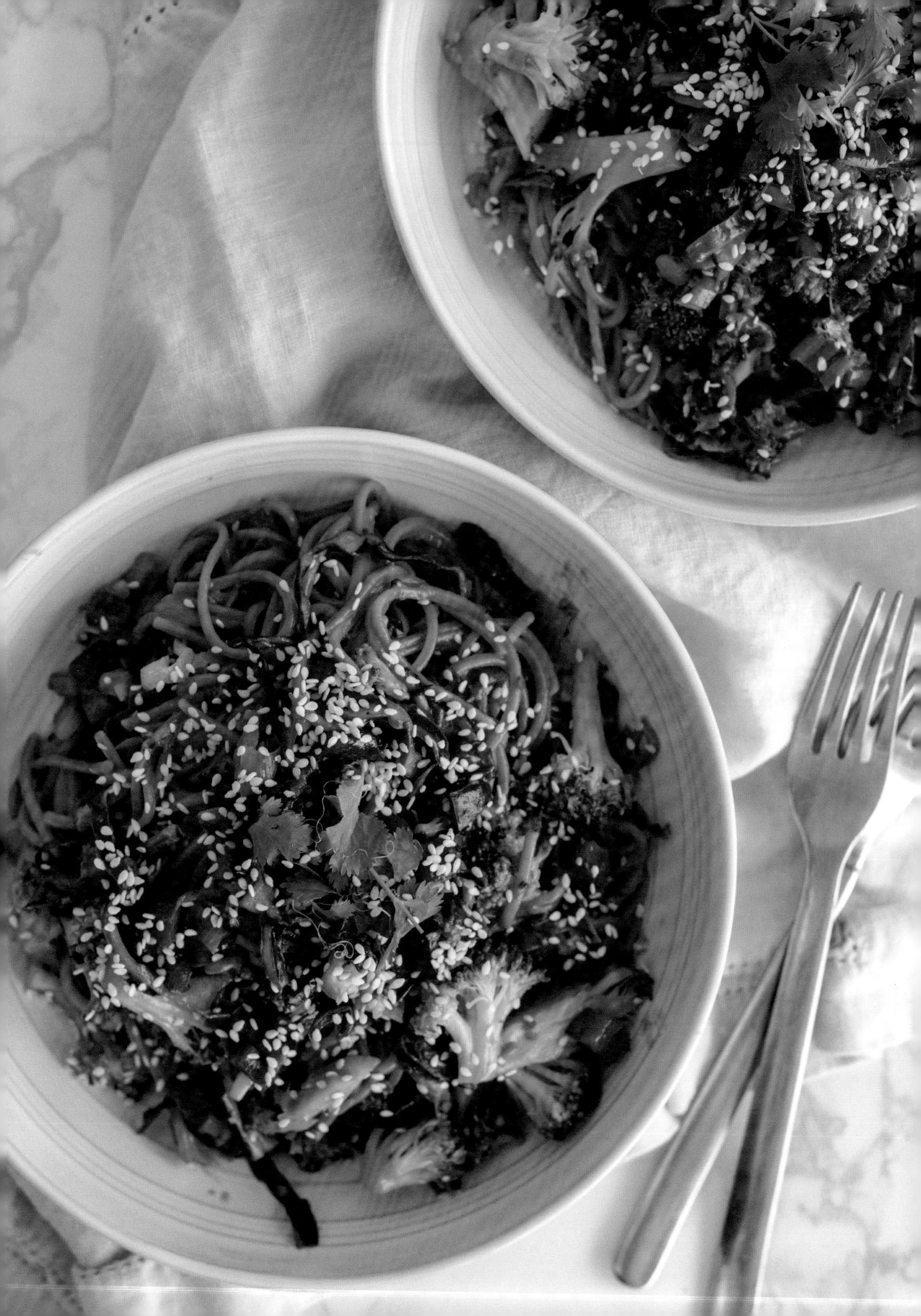

Cauliflower Tikka Masala

DAIRY-FREE | GLUTEN-FREE | VEGAN | NUT-FREE | VEGETARIAN

YIELDS 6 SERVINGS

Stir Fry Ingredients

1 Tbsp coconut oil
1 yellow onion, diced
4 cloves garlic, minced
1 inch ginger root, minced
1 red bell pepper, diced
2 cups cherry tomatoes, halved
1 can full-fat coconut milk
¼ cup no salt added tomato paste
1 Tbsp coconut sugar
¼ cup nutritional yeast
1 Tbsp garam masala
2 Tbsp paprika
1 tsp coriander
½ tsp black pepper
1 head cauliflower, chopped into florets
2 cups Indian basmati rice
Fresh cilantro, for topping

Sauce Directions

1. Heat the coconut oil in a medium-large pot on the stove.
2. Add in diced onion and minced garlic and let cook until the onions become translucent.
3. Add in minced ginger, tomatoes, tomato paste, bell pepper, spices, and coconut milk. (Basically, add in everything except for the cauliflower.)
4. Let the sauce simmer for 10 minutes, stirring occasionally. The tomatoes should cook down and the sauce should begin to thicken.
5. Add in chopped cauliflower and let simmer for 15 minutes, or until the cauliflower softens.
6. In a separate pot, or in a rice cooker, combine 2 cups of rice with 4 cups of water. Cook until the rice has absorbed the water and then take off of the heat and set aside.
7. Serve tikka masala with ½ cup rice and a generous amount of cauliflower tikka, and top with fresh cilantro leaves.

KCALS 453 | CARBOHYDRATE 64 G | PROTEIN 9 G | FAT 17 G | SATURATED FAT 14 G
SODIUM 261 MG | POTASSIUM 706 MG | FIBER 5 G | CALCIUM 61 MG
PHOSPHORUS 197 MG | IRON 4 MG

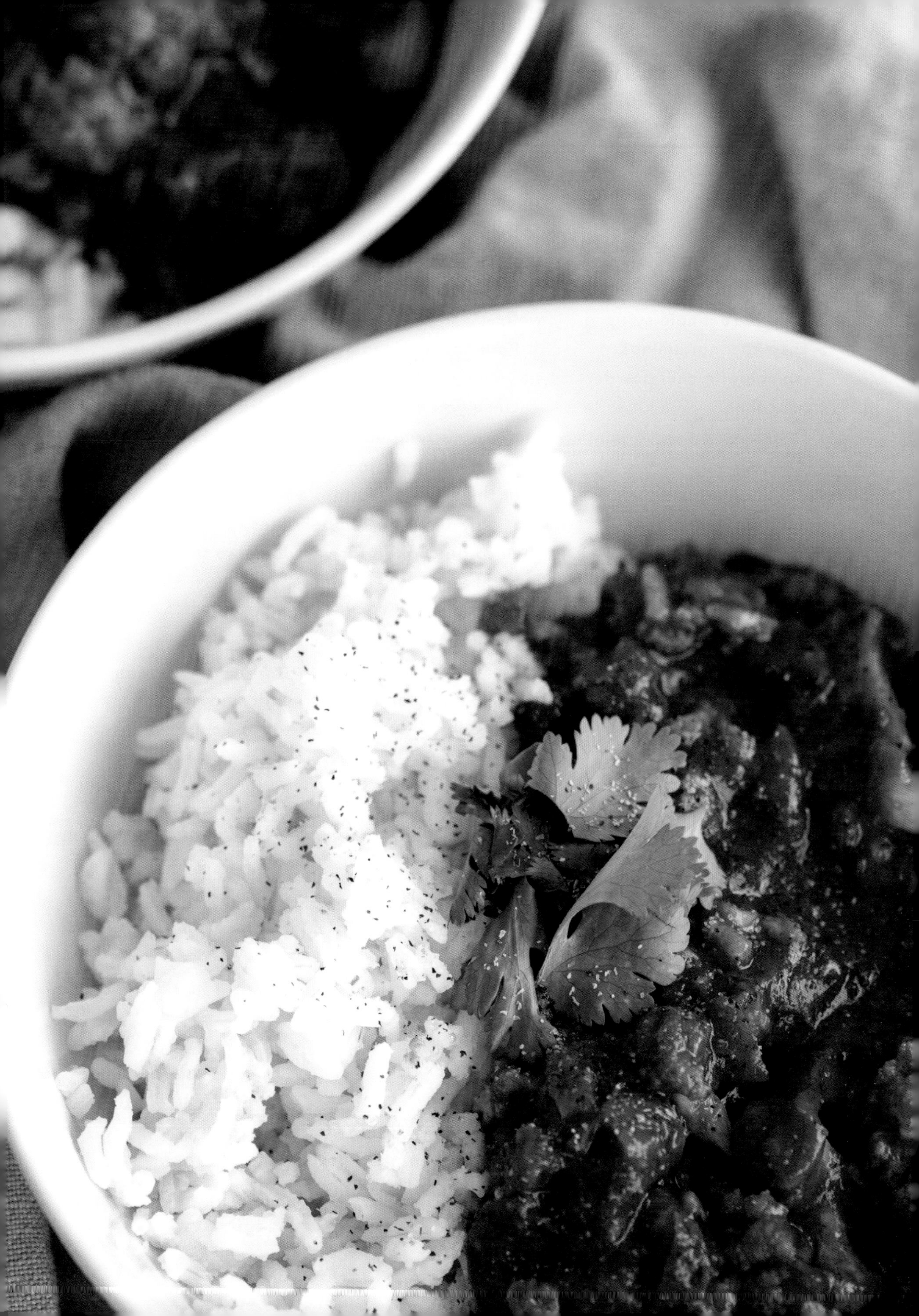

Smokey Tempeh Tacos

DAIRY-FREE | GLUTEN-FREE | VEGAN | VEGETARIAN

SERVES 4

Smokey Tempeh Ingredients

1 package of plain tempeh
2 Tbsp fresh lime juice
3 Tbsp pure maple syrup
3 Tbsp coconut aminos
1 tsp chipotle chili powder
1 tsp cumin
1 Tbsp olive oil

Cashew Chipotle Cream Ingredients

½ cup cashews
½ cup water (or more if needed)
2 Tbsp lime juice
1 Tbsp maple syrup
1 tsp smoked paprika
1 tsp cumin
1 clove garlic
½ tsp salt

Misc. Ingredients

8 corn tortillas
Peach pico (page 125)
Avocado (optional)

Smokey Tempeh Directions

1. Dice tempeh into small cubes and place to the side in a medium-sized bowl.
2. Add all other ingredients into a bowl and mix well.
3. Pour the marinade over the tempeh and let sit while you prepare the other toppings.
4. Once you have everything else ready for the tacos, pour tempeh and all the liquid marinade into a skillet over the stove. I like to cook mine until the sauce turns into a thick reduction and coats the tempeh. Tempeh does not necessarily have to be cooked for very long, so this should only take about 10 minutes.

Cashew Chipotle Cream Directions

1. Place all ingredients into a high-speed blender and blend on high until smooth.
2. Store in the refrigerator for up to 1 week.

Taco Assembly

1. Warm tortillas in the oven.
2. Add about ½ cup of tempeh.
3. Top with about 1/8 cup peach pico.
4. Add avocado or any other desired toppings.
5. Drizzle with your chipotle cream and enjoy!

KCALS 334 | CARBOHYDRATE 48 G | PROTEIN 14 G | FAT 12 G | SATURATED FAT 2 G
SODIUM 270 MG | POTASSIUM 364 MG | FIBER 1 G | CALCIUM 86 MG
PHOSPHORUS 155 MG | IRON 3 MG

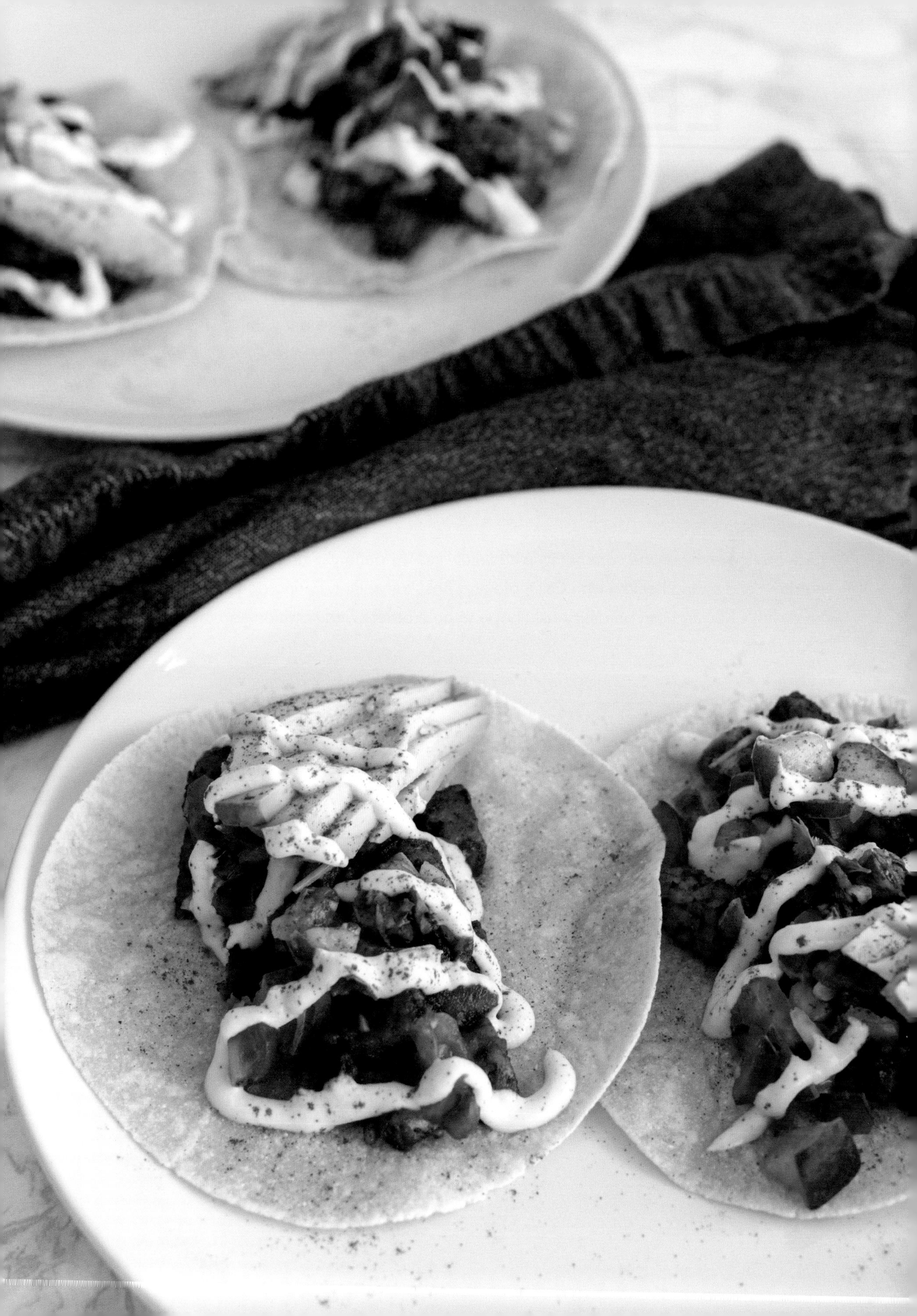

LENTIL SOUP

DAIRY-FREE I NUT-FREE I VEGAN I VEGETARIAN

SERVES 6

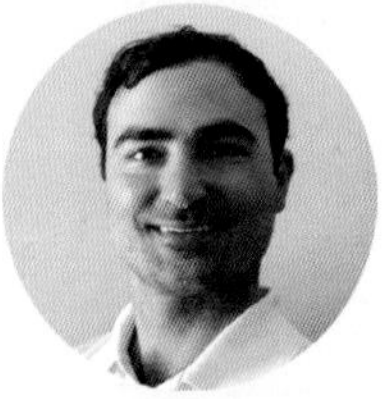

Hey there! My name is Anthony Valentine and I was diagnosed with IgA Nephropathy in April 2017. On January 31st, 2019, I was very blessed to have had my mother as my live donor for my kidney transplant. We both had great recoveries and my new kidney is doing really well.

With a degree in culinary arts & nutrition from the University of New Hampshire, my post-transplant CDK diet may have come a bit easier for me than it would for others. Which is why I've created the "cukebook" online recipe and nutrition community for people who have autoimmune diseases. (https://www.cukebook.org/)

I want to share my online community with fellow kidney patients, in hopes of helping with nutrition and eating healthy with CKD, pre and post-transplant. Eating doesn't have to be hard with CKD, and can be delicious! I hope to help others with nutrition and their CKD diets.

Ingredients

1 onion, chopped
1 carrot, large, chopped
2 celery ribs, chopped
2 garlic cloves, minced
½ cup brown lentils, dried, rinsed
½ cup crushed tomatoes
6 cups low sodium vegetable stock (or use water)
½ cup ditalini pasta, cooked al dente (or a gluten free pasta of choice)
2 bay leaves, dried
3 Tbsp olive oil
1½ tsp paprika powder, smoked
¼ tsp red pepper flakes (½ tsp if you like it a bit more spicy)
½ tsp salt, kosher

Directions

1. Add 3 tbsp of olive oil to a heavy-bottomed pot and turn to medium heat. When oil is hot, add onions, carrots, and celery and cook for 10-15 minutes or until translucent. Add garlic and red pepper flakes, cook for an additional 3-5 minutes.
2. Add vegetable stock, lentils, crushed tomatoes, bay leaves, paprika, and salt. Bring to a boil. Reduce to a low simmer, cover loosely, and cook for 30 minutes.
3. Remove bay leaves and pulse soup for 3-5 seconds using a stick blender. Simmer for an additional 20 minutes.
4. Mix in al dente pasta, cook for additional 1-2 minutes or until desired tenderness.
5. Serve with a fresh parsley sprig garnish.

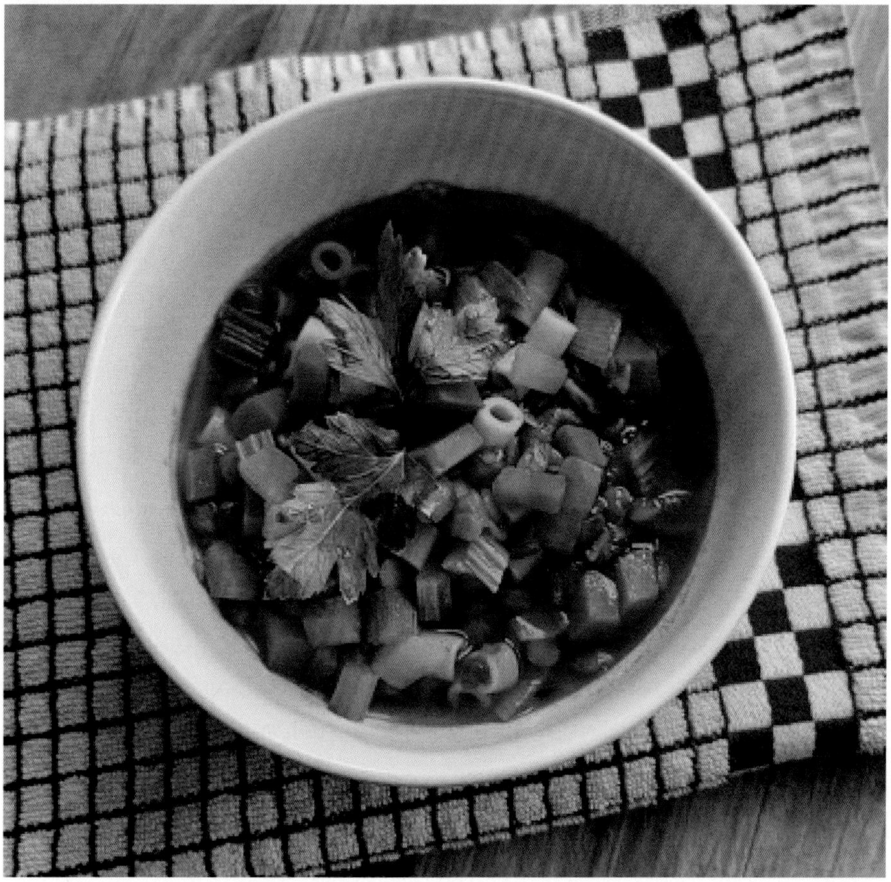

Lentil soup by Anthony Valentine

KCALS 164 | CARBOHYDRATE 19 G | PROTEIN 6 G | FAT 8 G | SATURATED FAT 1 G
SODIUM 258 MG | POTASSIUM 329 MG | FIBER 7 G | CALCIUM 43 MG
PHOSPHORUS 102 MG | IRON 2 MG

BITTER MELON STEW

DAIRY-FREE | GLUTEN-FREE | NUT-FREE | VEGAN | VEGETARIAN

SERVES 4

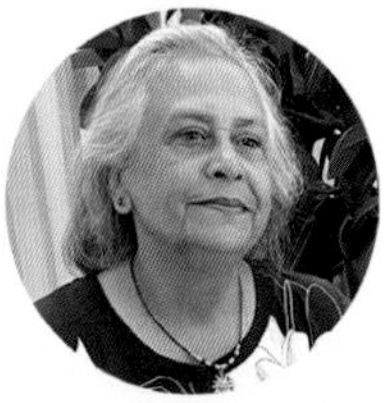

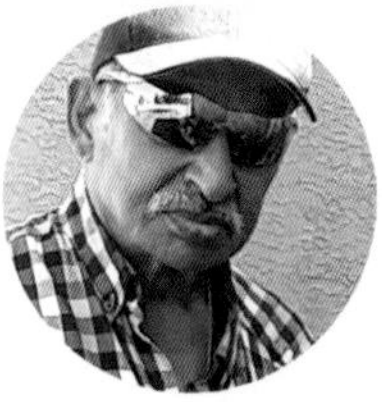

My husband, Dipten, and I are originally from West Bengal, a state in the eastern part of India. Canada has been our home for the past 45 years. Almost two years ago Dipten was diagnosed with IgA Nephropathy. We had never heard about this disease until the nephrologist talked about it. Fear robbed our ability to think as we listened to his diagnosis – IgAN is a rare kidney disease with no effective treatment. Then came the gloomy prediction that in two years Dipten's kidney function would deteriorate and he might need a transplant. He would, however, be too old to undergo such a complicated surgery said the doctor. Dipten was 71 at that time.

Those were dark days. We had no one to turn to for advice or encouragement. The local Kidney Foundation could not connect us with anyone who had IgAN. We tried to get as much information as possible through Google. While searching the web one day I found the IgA Nephropathy Foundation and reached out to Bonnie Schneider.

Bonnie replied quickly. Her story and positivity gave us much-needed hope. She was practical yet sensitive. Any time I contact her she is always there for us. Now the day is not too far when there will be effective medications for IgAN. In the meantime, Dipten must watch his blood pressure and control his diet. We eat Indian food daily. I cook the same dishes as my mother did but I have tweaked them so they are low in sodium and potassium.

In summer Bengalis (people from Bengal) generally prefer less spicy food that is easier on the stomach. Back in India, when the temperature outside rose, my mother prepared mixed vegetable stew with bitter melon. It was not my favourite vegetable when I was growing up. Since it is rich in vitamins, we had to eat it. The stew was always the first course of a meal (like soup or salad in North America). Until I finished the veggies that my mother put on my plate, I could not have the next course which was either fish or meat.

Moral of the story: it is an acquired taste and now I like bitter melon. We eat it often in Canada. As you can see on the ingredients list below, I used a ¼ teaspoon of salt only. Lemon juice and sugar are good substitutes. The dish will be slightly tangy which cuts down the bitterness of the melon. My mother never used lemon juice because our family was not on a restricted diet. Also, I did not use broccoli but you can if you like.

Small tip: if you have never tried bitter melon, use only half of one in the stew. Gradually you can increase the amount as your tastebuds get used to the bitterness. Ready to cook? Let's roll!

Ingredients

1/2 cup fresh green beans cut into 1-inch slices
1 medium bitter melon, seeds removed and diced (1/4-inch pieces)
1 large carrot, peeled and diced (1/2-inch pieces)
2 Chinese eggplants diced (3/4-inch pieces)
1 medium zucchini diced (3/4-inch pieces)
1 cup broccoli florets, chopped into smaller pieces (optional)
1 fresh green or red chili pepper cut in half (optional)
2 teaspoons olive oil
1 1/4 cups water
1/4 teaspoon nigella seeds (available in Indian or East Asian grocery stores)
1 teaspoon ginger grated
1/4 teaspoon turmeric powder
1/4 teaspoon sea salt
3/4 teaspoon sugar (as per taste)
juice of 1/2 medium lemon

Process

In a heavy pot heat olive oil. Add nigella seeds. Let it sizzle. Lower heat to medium high and add bitter melon. Keep stirring to brown them a little. Add all other vegetables along with the chili and stir for about five minutes. Put turmeric and add 1/4 cup of water to prevent the spice from burning. Stir for about three minutes until the raw smell of turmeric goes away. Add a cup of water, salt and sugar. Turn up heat and let it boil. Put grated ginger; cover and cook for about ten minutes. When the veggies have softened add lemon juice. Taste the sauce. You may need a little more sugar or more lemon juice. Sauce should not be watery. It should coat the veggies nicely. Serve with steamed basmati rice.

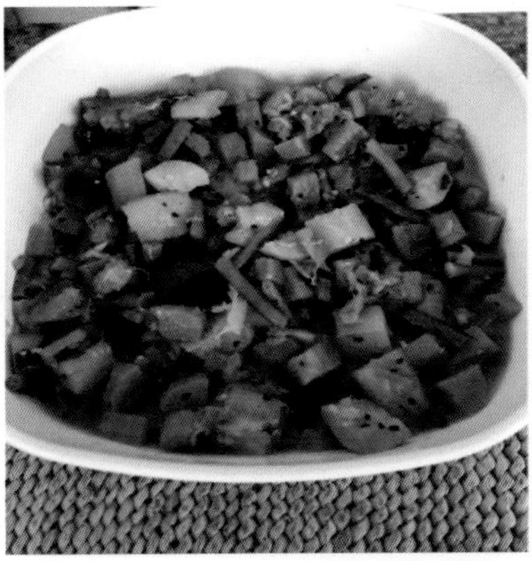

Bitter melon Stew by Dipti Chakravorty

KCALS 88 | CARBOHYDRATE 16 G | PROTEIN 3 G | FAT 3 G | SATURATED FAT 1 G
SODIUM 175 MG | POTASSIUM 666 MG | FIBER 6 G | CALCIUM 50 MG
PHOSPHORUS 85 MG | IRON 1 MG

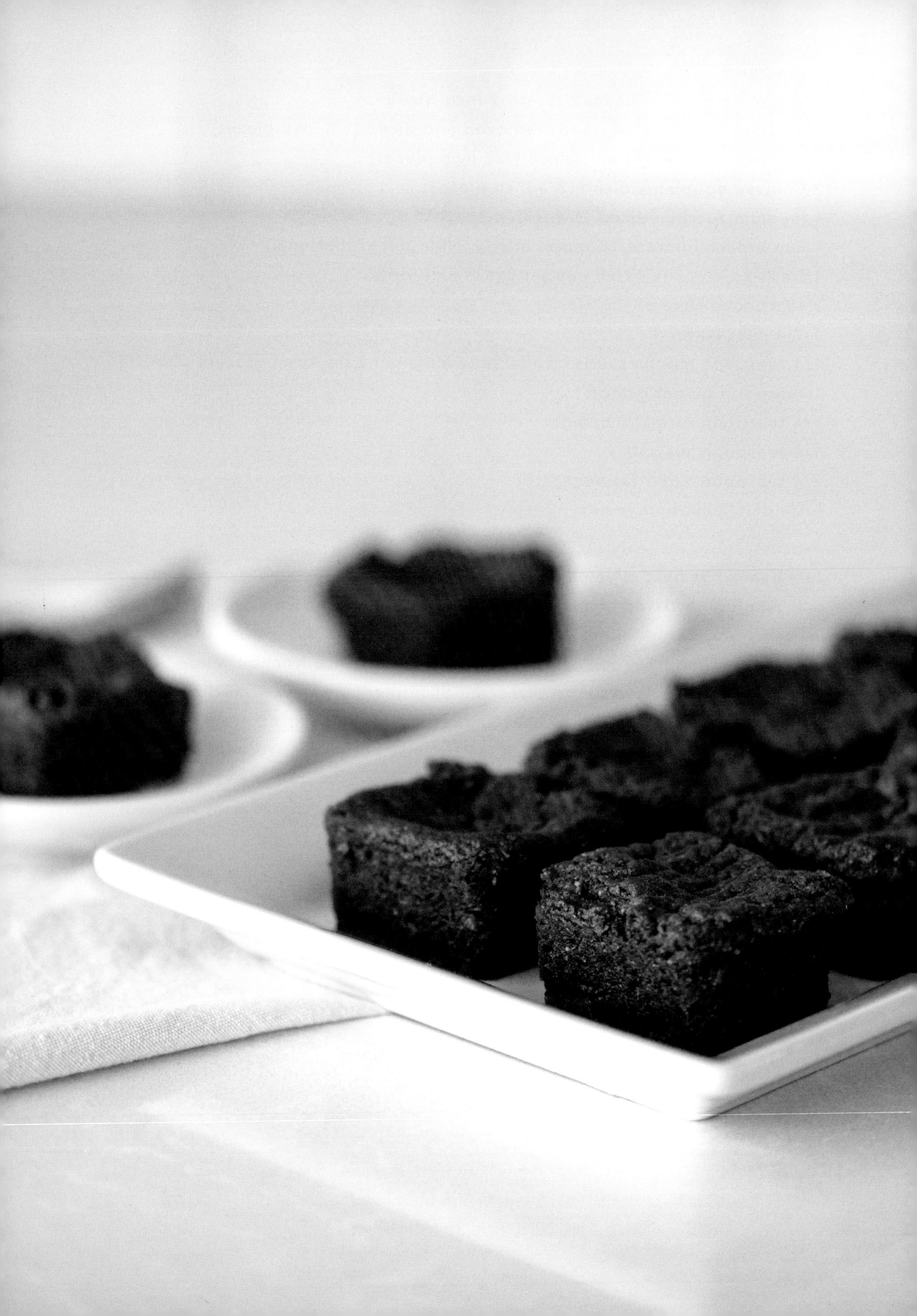

SNACKS & APPETIZERS

Granola

DAIRY-FREE | GLUTEN-FREE | VEGAN | VEGETARIAN

YIELDS 20 1/4-CUP SERVINGS

Ingredients

3 cups oats
1 cup sliced almonds
1 Tbsp cinnamon
½ cup pumpkin seeds
½ cup coconut flakes
½ tsp salt (or omit completely)
1 Tbsp vanilla extract
¼ cup pure maple syrup

Directions

1. Mix all ingredients in a medium-sized mixing bowl until well combined.
2. Bake at 350°F for 15–20 minutes or until golden brown.
3. Store in an air-tight container for up to 30 days.

CUSTOMIZE IT!
You can subsitute the almonds for any nut of your choice.

KCALS 114 | CARBOHYDRATE 13 G | PROTEIN 3 G | FAT 6 G | SATURATED FAT 2 G
SODIUM 60 MG | POTASSIUM 120 MG | FIBER 3 G | CALCIUM 31 MG
PHOSPHORUS 100 MG | IRON 1 MG

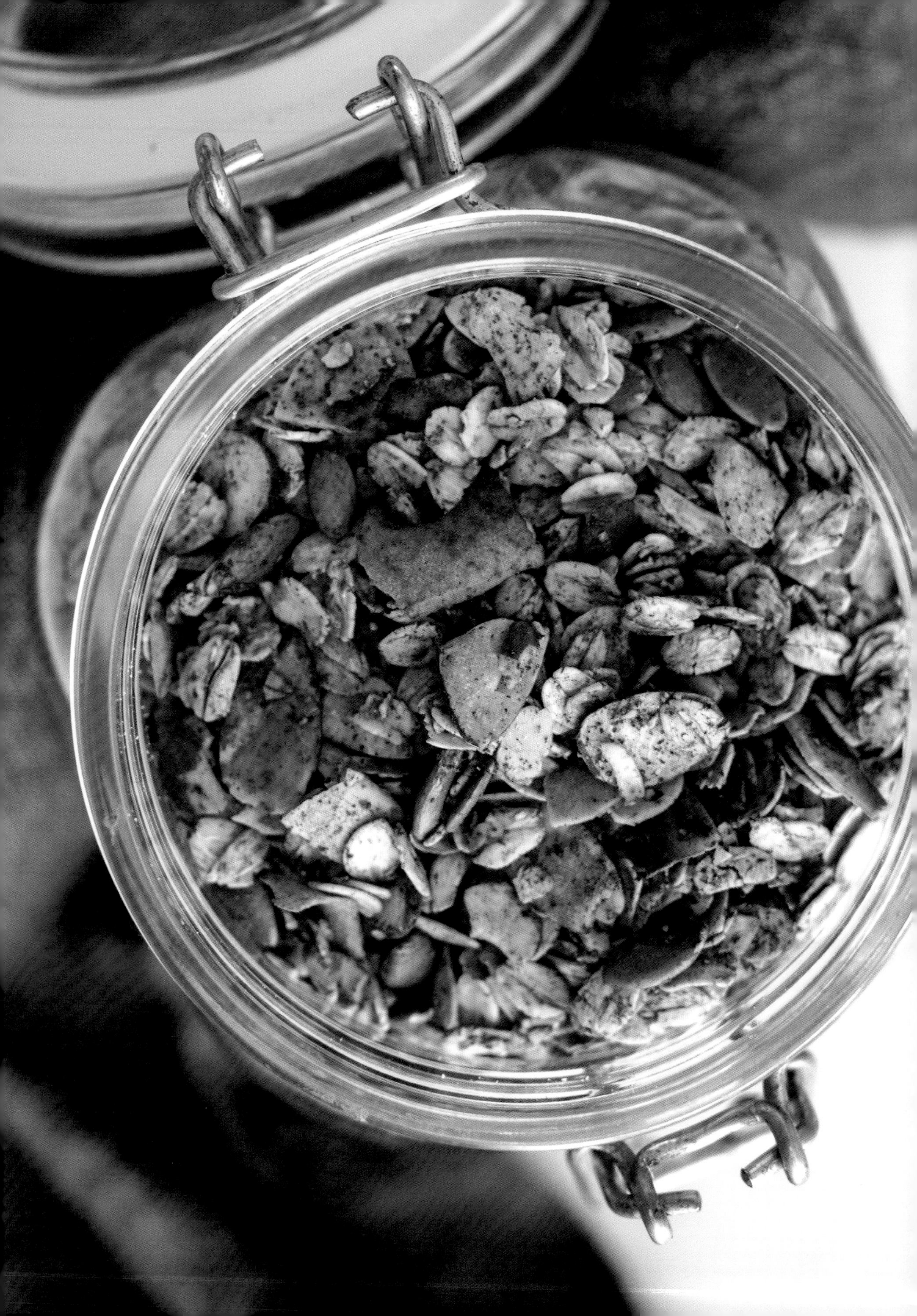

Energy Bars

DAIRY-FREE I GLUTEN-FREE I VEGAN I VEGETARIAN

YIELDS 12 BARS

Ingredients

1 cup rolled oats
½ cup cashew butter (sugar free)
1/8 cup flaxseed meal
1 Tbsp chia seeds
2/3 cup toasted coconut flakes
½ cup dark chocolate chips
1/3 cup honey
1 tsp vanilla extract
Pinch of salt

Directions

1. Line an 8x8 or 9x9 baking pan with parchment paper.
2. Add all ingredients into a mixing bowl and stir until well combined. It should feel like a very thick dough.
3. Place the dough into the baking pan and spread it out evenly. You may wish to use your hands to press it down firmly.
4. Place pan in the refrigerator for about 2 hours or the freezer for about 1 hour. Once it has firmed up, cut into 12 squares and keep in the refrigerator for up to 3 weeks or the freezer for up to 8 weeks.

These make for great snacks on the go or for a sweet treat! Kids love them too!

PRO TIP
Use local honey if possible!

KCALS 187 | CARBOHYDRATE 20 G | PROTEIN 4 G | FAT 11 G | SATURATED FAT 5 G
SODIUM 7 MG | POTASSIUM 131 MG | FIBER 2 G | CALCIUM 20 MG
PHOSPHORUS 106 MG | IRON 1 MG

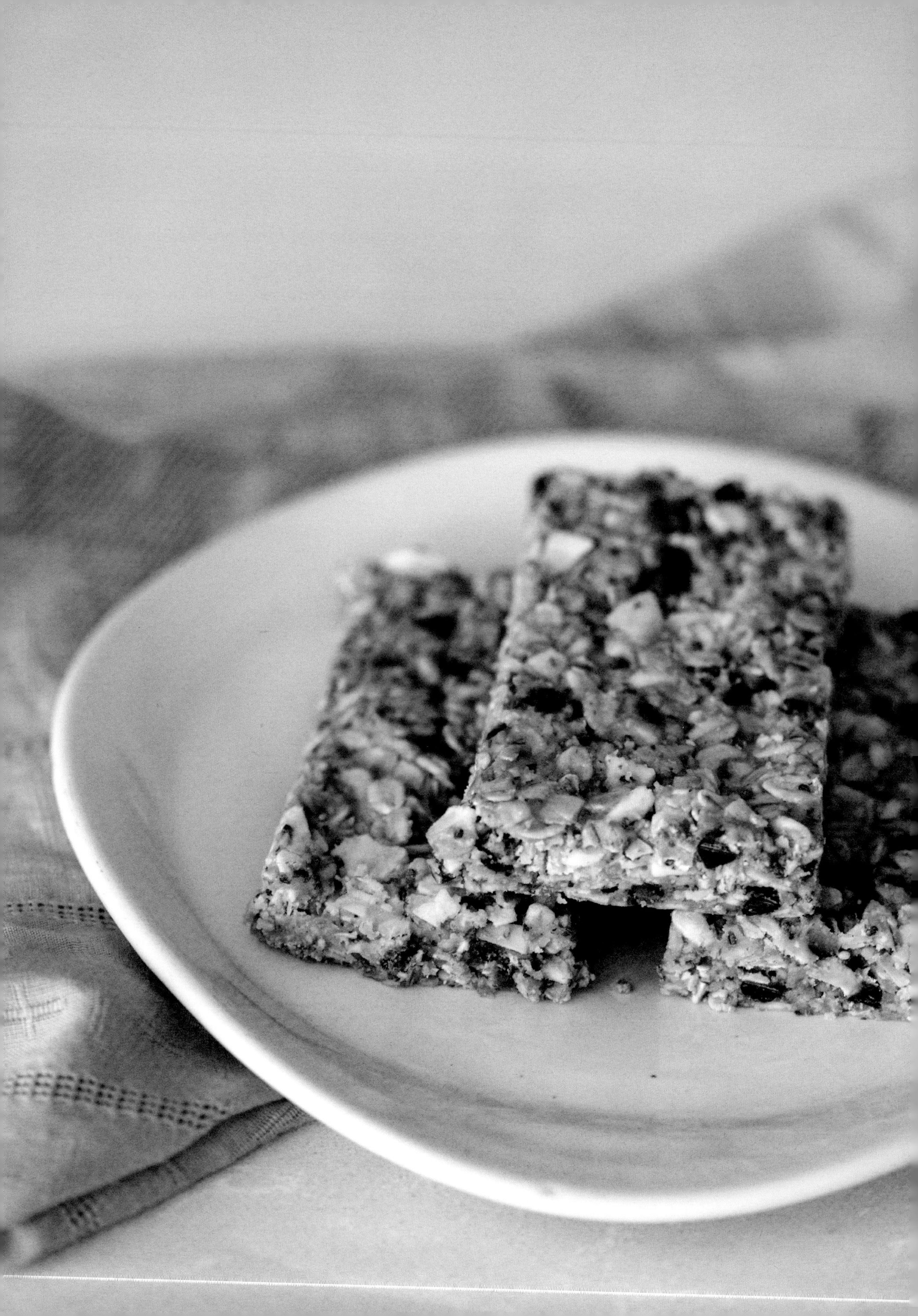

Hummus

DAIRY-FREE | GLUTEN-FREE | VEGAN | VEGETARIAN

YIELDS 2.5 CUPS / 10 SERVINGS

Ingredients

2 cups cooked chickpeas

½ cup tahini

½ cup olive oil

2 oz lemon juice

2 garlic cloves

½ tsp salt

1 tsp smoked paprika

1 tsp ground cumin

Directions

1. Place all ingredients in a food processor and blend until smooth and creamy.
2. Store in an airtight container in the refrigerator for up to 10 days.

OIL FREE?
Simply substitute water in place of olive oil.

KCALS 214 | CARBOHYDRATE 10 G | PROTEIN 5 G | FAT 18 G | SATURATED FAT 2 G
SODIUM 136 MG | POTASSIUM 171 MG | FIBER 3 G | CALCIUM 70 MG
PHOSPHORUS 89 MG | IRON 2 MG

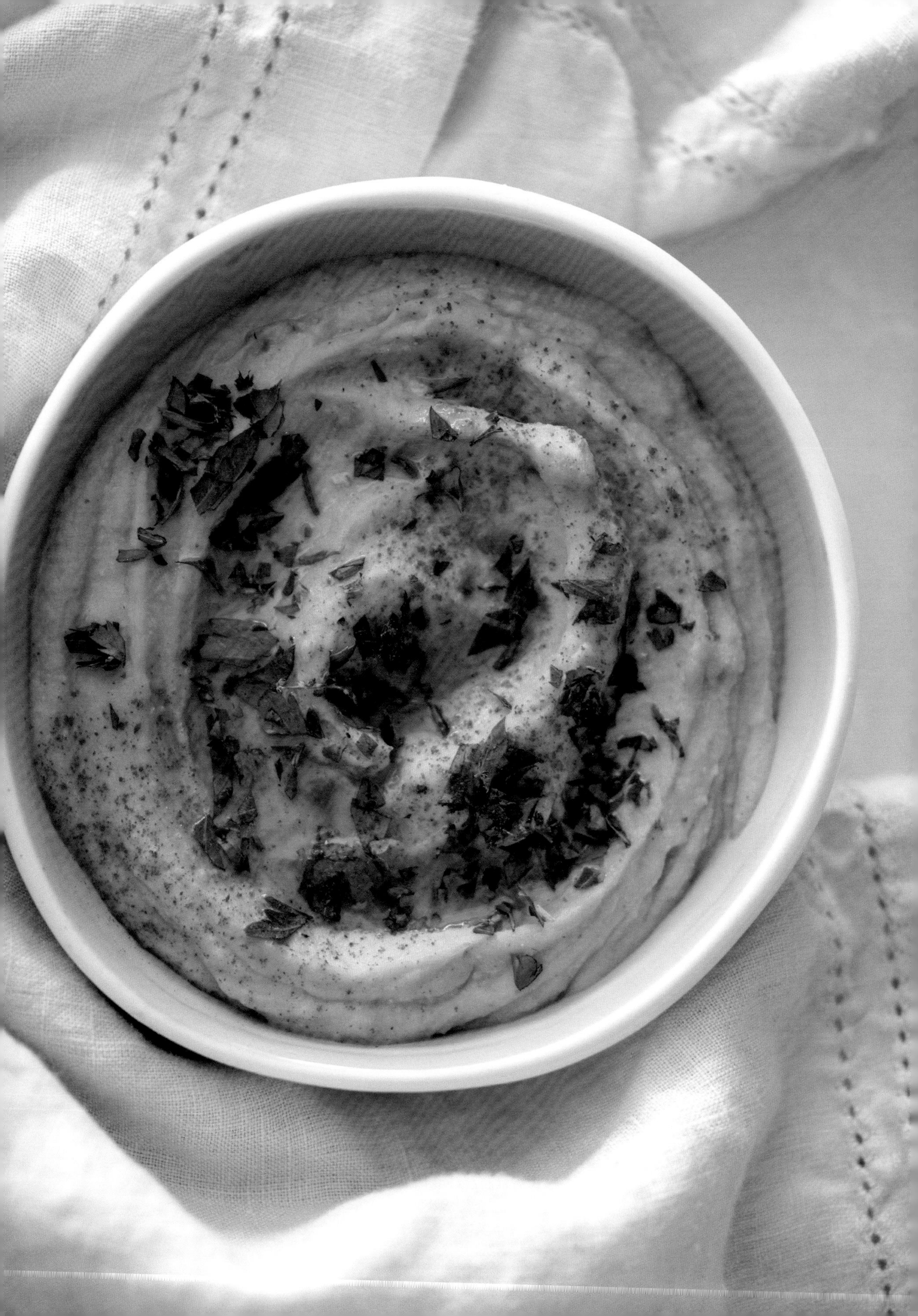

Cashew Queso

DAIRY-FREE I GLUTEN-FREE I VEGAN I VEGETARIAN

YIELDS ABOUT 1 CUP / 10 SERVINGS

Ingredients

1 cup cashews

2 Tbsp nutritional yeast

1 cup water

1½ Tbsp fresh lemon juice

½ tsp salt

1 tsp smoked paprika

1 tsp chili powder

1 garlic clove

Directions

1. Place all ingredients in a blender and blend until smooth and creamy.
2. Store in an airtight container in the refrigerator for up to 7 days.
3. Serve with roasted vegetables, corn chips, or gluten-free tortillas.

KCALS 79 | CARBOHYDRATE 5 G | PROTEIN 3 G | FAT 6 G | SATURATED FAT 1 G
SODIUM 122 MG | POTASSIUM 127 MG | FIBER 1 G | CALCIUM 7 MG
PHOSPHORUS 78 MG | IRON 1 MG

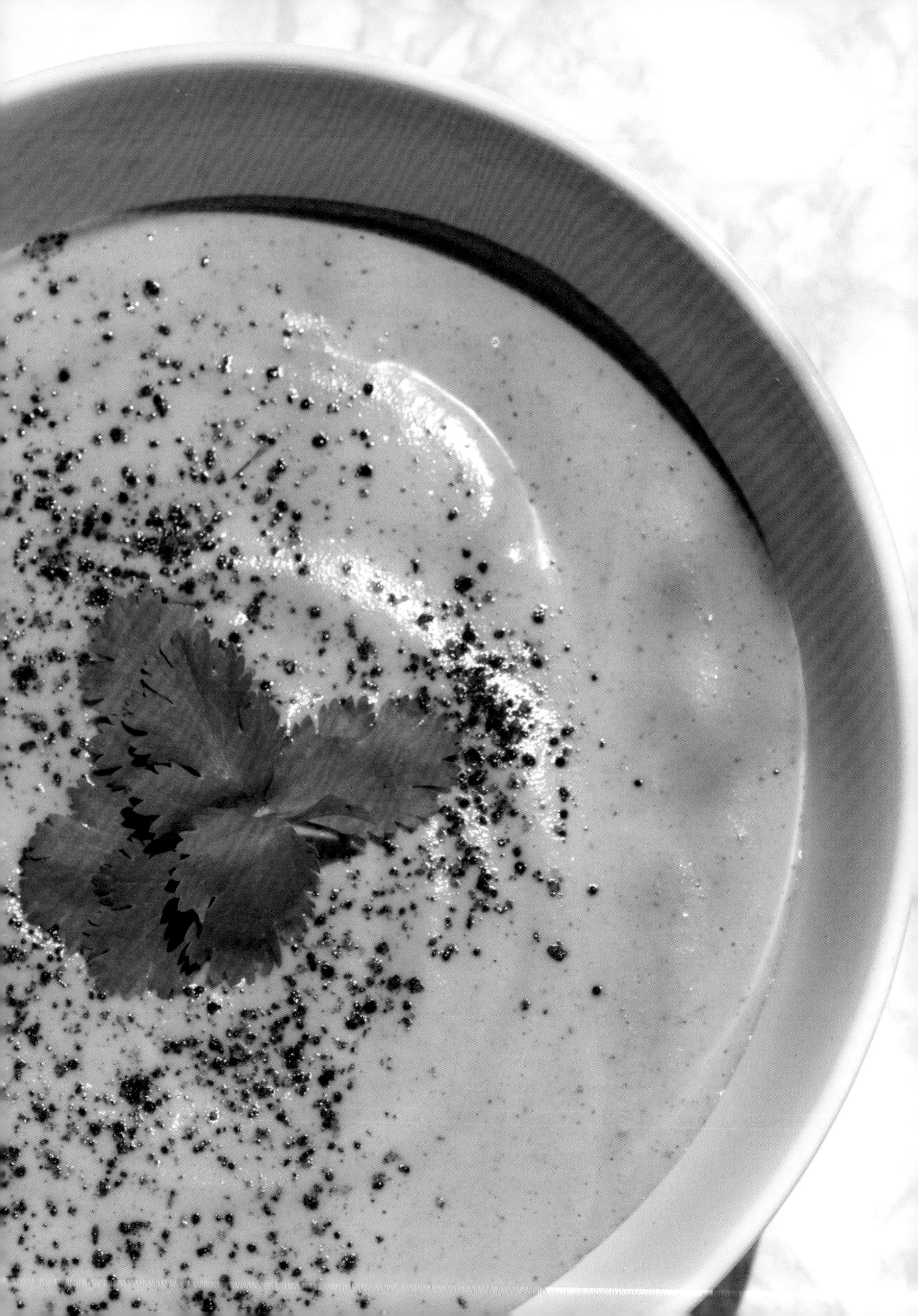

Peach Pico

DAIRY-FREE | GLUTEN-FREE | VEGAN | NUT-FREE | VEGETARIAN

YIELDSVV ABOUT 2 CUPS / 4 SERVINGS

Ingredients

1 ripe peach, diced
½ red onion, diced
1 small red bell pepper, diced
1 tomato, diced
¼ cup fresh cilantro, chopped
¼ cup fresh basil, chopped
1 jalapeño, diced
2 Tbsp fresh lime juice

Directions

1. Add all of your chopped ingredients into a large bowl and toss well.
2. Serve immediately with cashew queso, corn chips, or gluten-free tortillas.
3. Store in an airtight container in the refrigerator for up to 7 days.

KCALS 25 | CARBOHYDRATE 6 G | PROTEIN 1 G | FAT 1 G | SATURATED FAT 1 G
SODIUM 6 MG | POTASSIUM 153 MG | FIBER 1 G | CALCIUM 10 MG
PHOSPHORUS 21 MG | IRON 1 MG

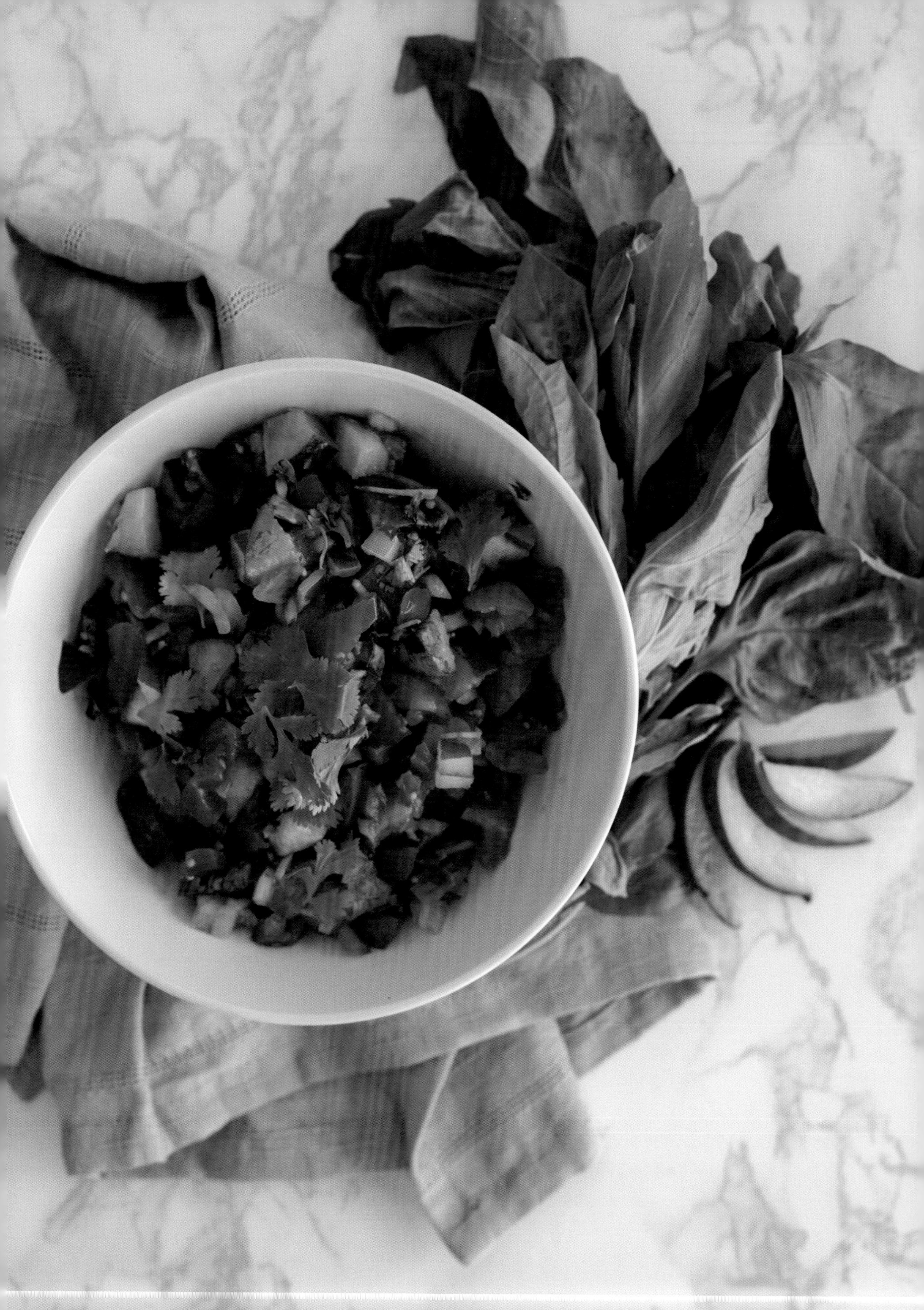

Kale Chips

DAIRY-FREE | GLUTEN-FREE | VEGAN | NUT-FREE | VEGETARIAN

YIELDS ABOUT 3 CUPS / 6 SERVINGS

Ingredients

8 cups curly kale, de-stemmed (about one bundle)
¼ cup olive oil
½ tsp salt
1 tsp black pepper
3 Tbsp nutritional yeast

Directions

1. Preheat oven to 350°F.
2. Add all chopped ingredients into a large bowl and toss well. Kale should feel well coated.
3. Bake for 12 minutes and then remove from the oven and toss around gently. If they are not fully crispy, you can bake them for an additional 4 minutes.
4. Remove from oven, let cool, and store in an airtight container.

KCALS 115 | CARBOHYDRATE 5 G | PROTEIN 3 G | FAT 10 G | SATURATED FAT 8 G
SODIUM 108 MG | POTASSIUM 336 MG | FIBER 4 G | CALCIUM 229 MG
PHOSPHORUS 50 MG | IRON 2 MG

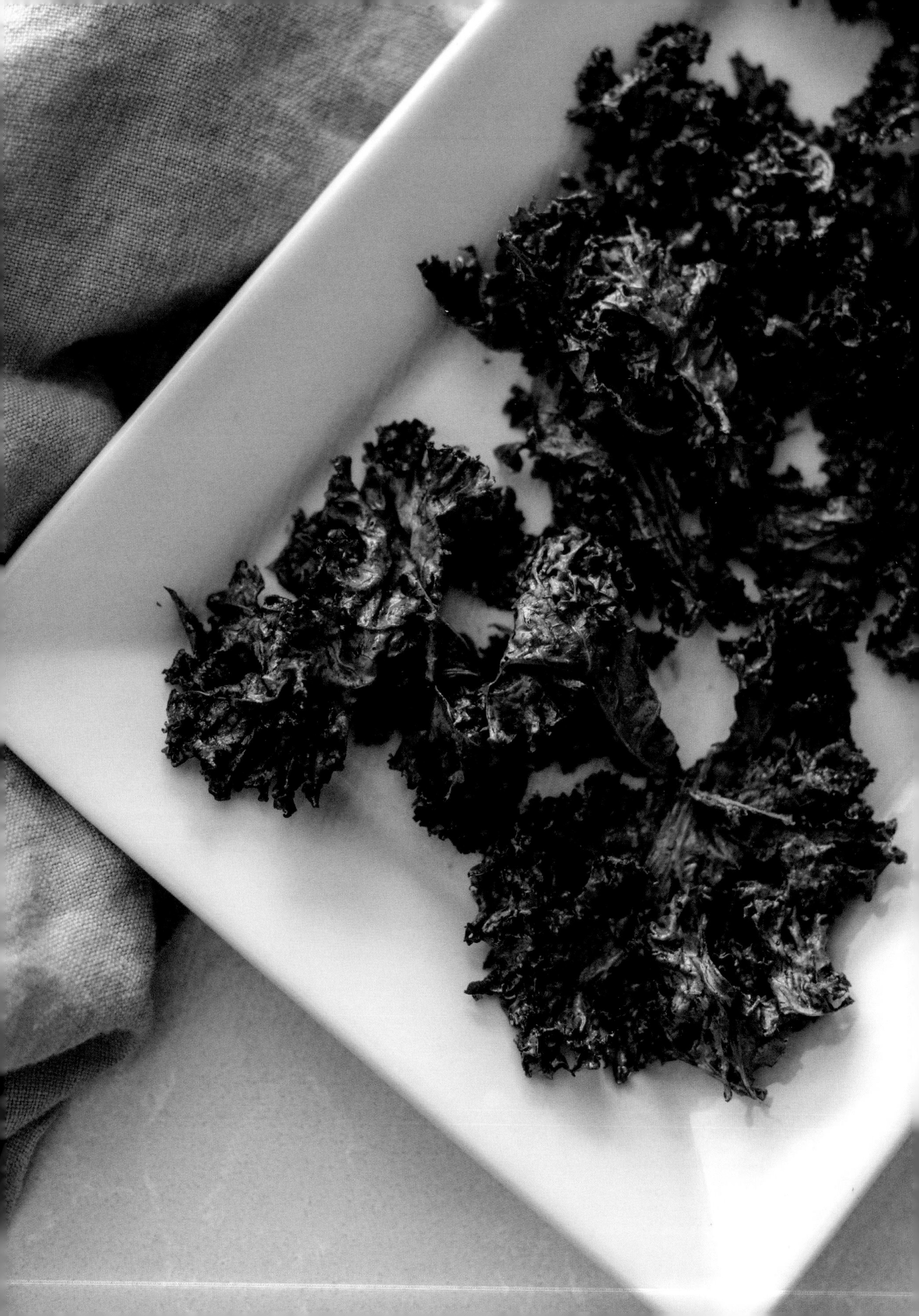

AIR FRYER ARTICHOKE HEARTS

DAIRY-FREE | NUT-FREE | VEGAN | VEGETARIAN

SERVES 6

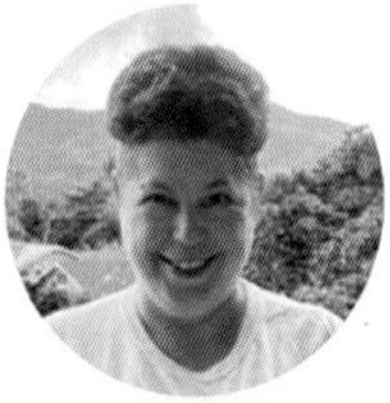

In August 2019, my life changed as I was diagnosed with IgA Nephropathy through a kidney biopsy. At the time, my eGFR was 22, and I had a creatinine of 2.5. My nephrologist put me on high doses of prednisone, and I was given a plan to reduce my protein leakage through the prescribed medication, fish oil and diet changes. I also attended a 6-week course about living with Chronic Kidney Disease. Through this class it became clear that I was being prepped for dialysis.

Determined to not go on dialysis, I became committed to making whatever life changes I needed to make. The big one was deciding to go plant based. As a person who worked and lived a food service lifestyle, this was a major life change. As I drove deeper into the new diet, I found myself missing my favorite dishes. I decided to start creating and making my own recipes of my favorite dishes, but with a plant-based spin.

Now after following a strict plant based, low sodium diet, paired with medications and supplements, I am considered stable with an eGFR base line of 40 to 45, and a creatinine around 1.4.

I created these artichoke wings as a play on chicken wings, packed with flavor. They turned out great, and even my meat-eating family members enjoyed them. These can be served as a main with some pasta, as an appetizer dipped in some vegan buffalo sauce or vegan ranch, or as a filling for tacos or burritos.

- Judy Atkin

Ingredients

12 oz frozen artichoke hearts
1 cup veganaise (or any vegan mayonnaise)
¼ cup fresh lemon juice
2 cups panko (low sodium)
2 Tbsp nutritional yeast
2 tsp Italian seasoning
1 tsp Aleppo pepper
1 tsp garlic powder

Directions

1. In a shallow bowl mix veganaise and lemon juice.
2. In another shallow bowl, combine the panko, nutritional yeast and seasonings.
3. Dredge artichoke in the veganaise mixture, and then into the dried mix.
4. Cook in an air fryer at 375°F for 10 minutes.

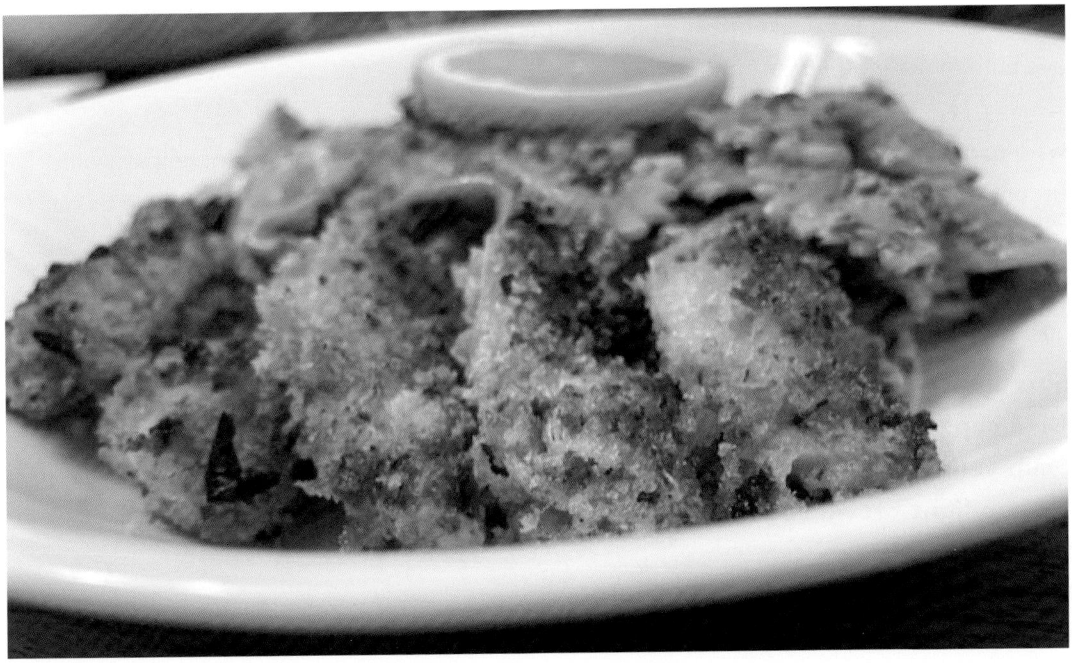

Air Fryer Artichoke Hearts by Judy Atkin

KCALS 284 | CARBOHYDRATE 47 G | PROTEIN 7 G | FAT 9 G | SATURATED FAT 1 G
SODIUM 405 MG | POTASSIUM 184 MG | FIBER 6 G | CALCIUM 19 MG
PHOSPHORUS 45 MG | IRON 1 MG

CORNBREAD

DAIRY-FREE I NUT-FREE I VEGAN I VEGETARIAN

SERVES 8

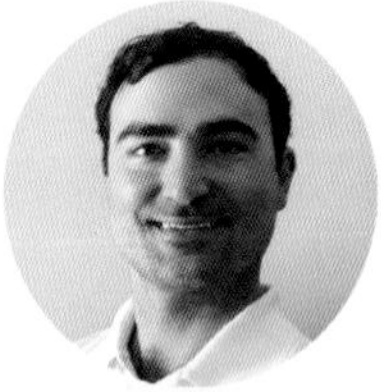

Hey there! My name is Anthony Valentine and I was diagnosed with IgA Nephropathy in April 2017. On January 31st, 2019, I was very blessed to have had my mother as my live donor for my kidney transplant. We both had great recoveries and my new kidney is doing really well.

With a degree in culinary arts & nutrition from the University of New Hampshire, my post-transplant CDK diet may have come a bit easier for me than it would for others. Which is why I've created the "cukebook" online recipe and nutrition community for people who have autoimmune diseases. (https://www.cukebook.org/)

I want to share my online community with fellow kidney patients, in hopes of helping with nutrition and eating healthy with CKD, pre and post-transplant. Eating doesn't have to be hard with CKD, and can be delicious! I hope to help others with nutrition and their CKD diets.

Ingredients

1-1/4 cups all purpose flour (or a gluten free flour)
1 cup yellow corn meal
2/3 cup light brown sugar
1-1/2 cup oat milk
1/3 cup canola oil (or oil of choice)
1 tbsp salt-free baking powder
1/4 tsp cayenne pepper
1/4 tsp kosher salt

Directions

1. **Preheat the oven to 450 °F and lightly grease a 9 x 13 pan.**
2. **In a large bowl, mix together the flour, cornmeal, sugar, cayenne pepper, salt, and baking powder.**
3. **Add oat milk and canola oil to the bowl with the dry ingredients. Stir until well combined.**
4. **Pour batter into greased pan**

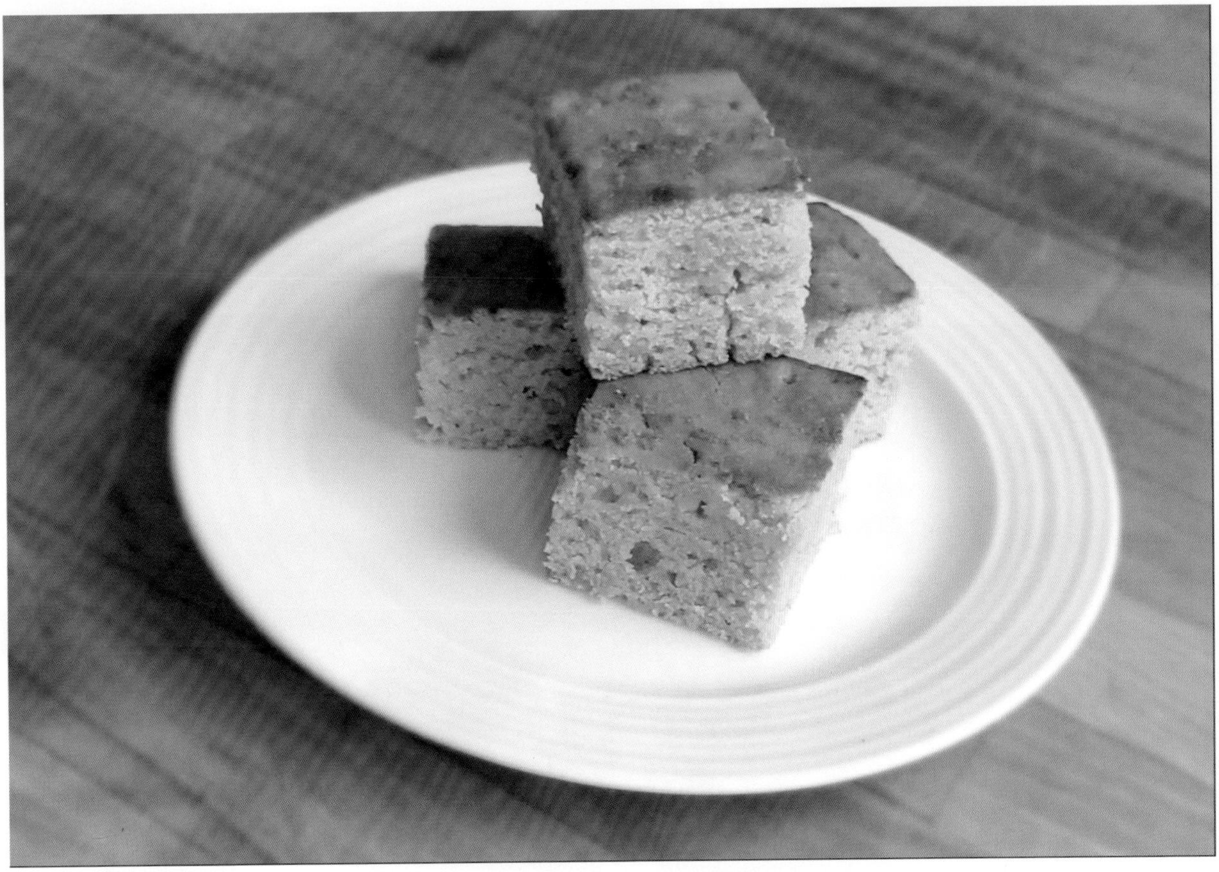

Cornbread by Anthony Valentine

KCALS 171 | CARBOHYDRATE 28 G | PROTEIN 2 G | FAT 6 G | SATURATED FAT 1 G
SODIUM 52 MG | POTASSIUM 149 MG | FIBER 1 G | CALCIUM 73 MG
PHOSPHORUS 90 MG | IRON 1 MG

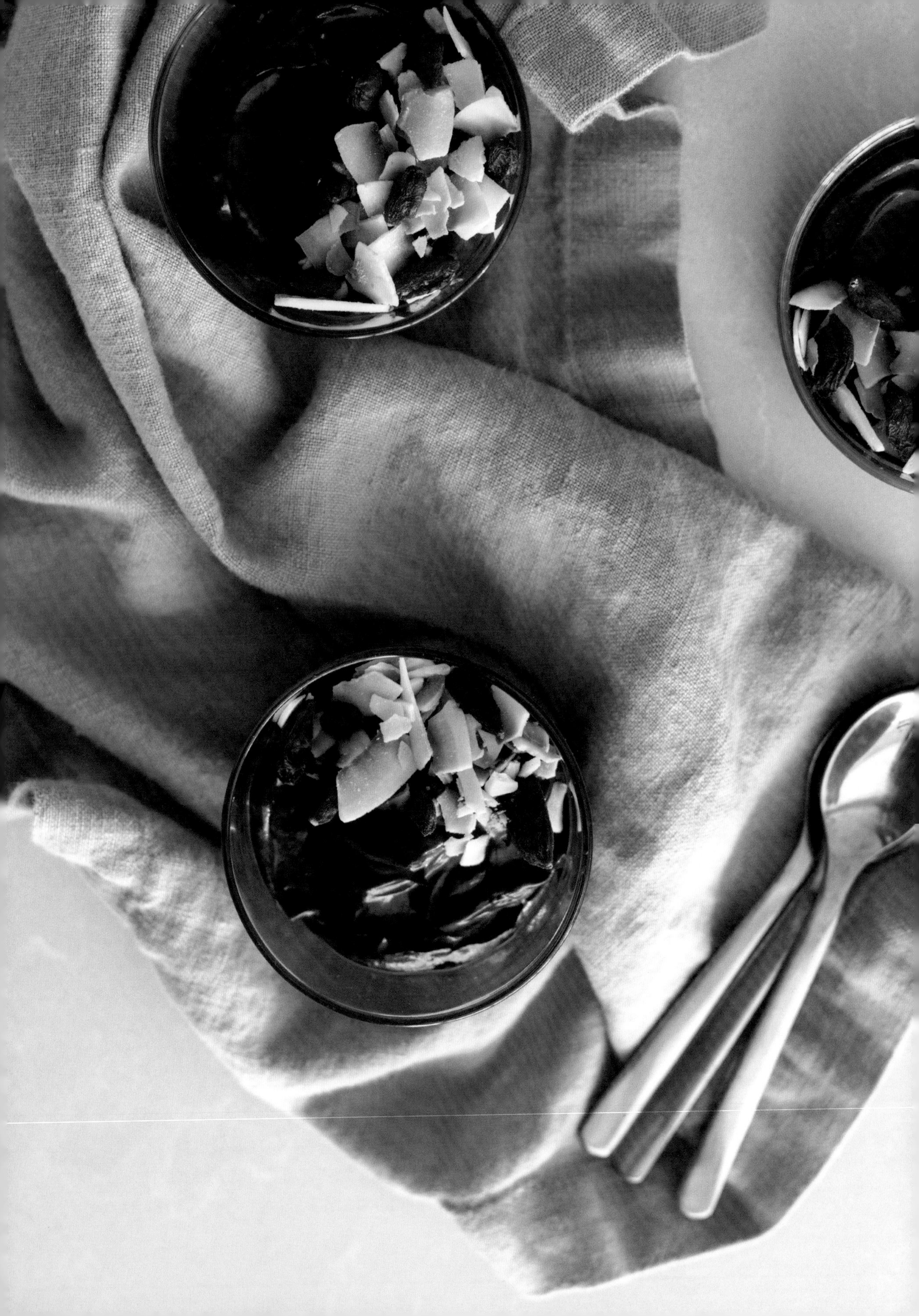

DESSERTS

20-Minute Oatmeal Chocolate Chip Cookies

DAIRY-FREE | GLUTEN-FREE | VEGAN | VEGETARIAN

YIELDS 12 COOKIES

Ingredients

½ cup creamy almond butter
½ cup pure maple syrup
1 tsp vanilla extract
½ tsp ground cinnamon
½ tsp salt
¾ cup whole oats
¼ cup oat flour
3 Tbsp almond flour
½ cup non-dairy dark chocolate chips

Directions

1. Preheat oven to 350°F.
2. Mix all ingredients in a mixing bowl.
3. Scoop/form small balls and place on a lined or nonstick baking sheet.
4. Bake for 10–12 minutes until slightly golden brown.

Feel free to substitute almond butter for cashew butter or peanut butter if preferred.

KCALS 143 | CARBOHYDRATE 18 G | PROTEIN 3 G | FAT 7 G | SATURATED FAT 1 G
SODIUM 101 MG | POTASSIUM 136 MG | FIBER 2 G | CALCIUM 55 MG
PHOSPHORUS 85 MG | IRON 1 MG

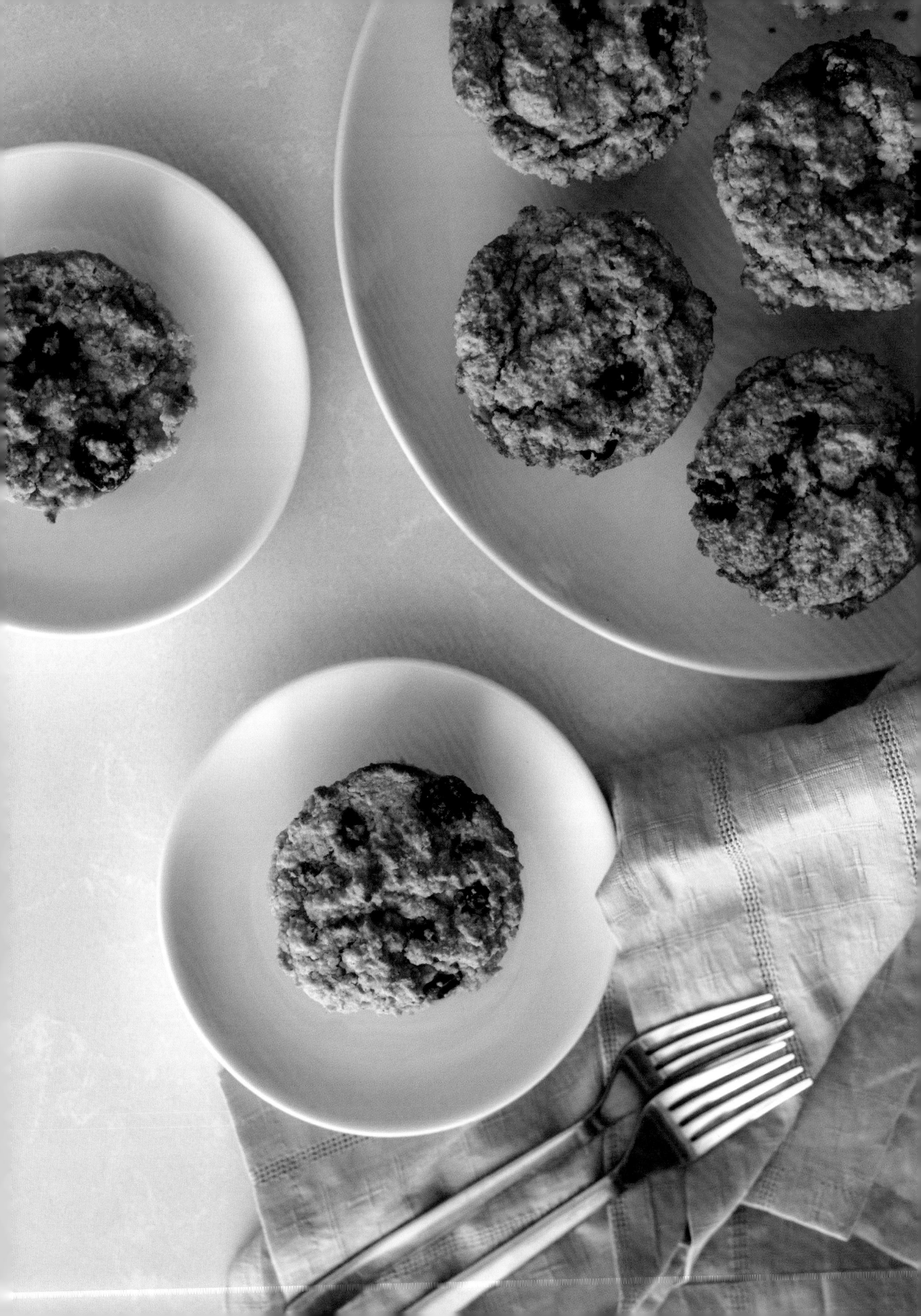

Almond Butter Brownies

DAIRY-FREE | GLUTEN-FREE | VEGAN | VEGETARIAN

YIELDS 12–16 BROWNIES

Ingredients

2 cups almond butter
4 Tbsp flaxseed mixed with
8 Tbsp water (or 2 eggs)
1 cup coconut sugar
1 cup dark chocolate chips
1 tsp vanilla extract
1 tsp baking soda
½ tsp sea salt

Directions

1. Preheat oven to 350°F.
2. Combine the flaxseed and water in a small cup or bowl and stir well, then set aside.
3. Grease a small 8x8 square pan with coconut oil or line with parchment paper, then set aside.
4. Combine all ingredients except for chocolate chips in a large mixing bowl. Mix well.
5. Add in the chocolate chips and stir again.
6. Place the batter in your square pan and spread out evenly.
7. Bake 20–30 minutes until golden brown, or until a toothpick comes out clean.
8. Let the brownies cool for at least 10–15 minutes before cutting.
9. Enjoy!

KCALS 300 | CARBOHYDRATE 20 G | PROTEIN 8 G | FAT 23 G | SATURATED FAT 4 G
SODIUM 166 MG | POTASSIUM 136 MG | FIBER 2 G | CALCIUM 55 MG
PHOSPHORUS 85 MG | IRON 1 MG

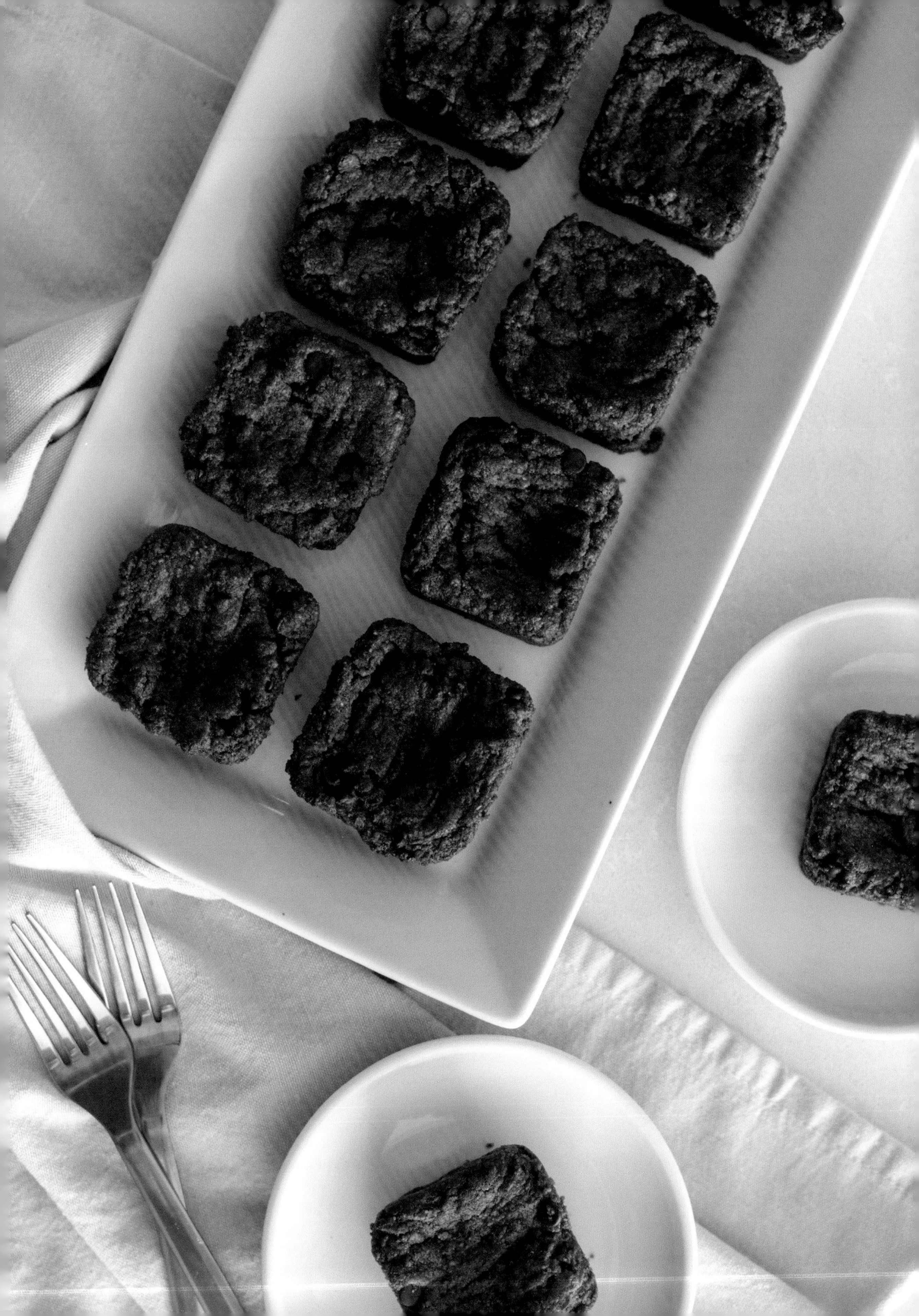

Apple Crisp

DAIRY-FREE I GLUTEN-FREE I VEGAN I VEGETARIAN

YIELDS 6 -8 SERVINGS

Filling Ingredients

4 medium apples
½ oz lemon juice
1/3 cup coconut sugar
¾ tsp ground cinnamon
1½ Tbsp arrowroot starch
2 Tbsp water
¼ tsp ground ginger
1 pinch nutmeg

Topping Ingredients

½ cup gluten-free rolled oats
¼ cup almond flour
¼ cup oat flour
½ cup coconut sugar
¼ cup pecans, roughly chopped
½ tsp ground cinnamon
¼ cup melted coconut oil

Directions

1. Preheat oven to 350°F.
2. Peel apples, quarter, remove cores, and use a paring knife to thinly slice lengthwise.
3. Add apples to a large mixing bowl and toss with remaining filling ingredients. Toss until well combined. Pour into an 8x8 baking dish.
4. Rinse and wipe out mixing bowl and add all topping ingredients. Stir to combine. Pour the topping over the apples in an even layer.
5. Bake for 50 minutes to 1 hour (uncovered) or until the filling is bubbly, the apples are very fork tender (especially in the center of the dish), and the topping is deep golden brown.
6. Let rest at least 30 minutes before serving. This is delicious served with vanilla non-dairy ice cream.

KCALS 243 | CARBOHYDRATE 37 G | PROTEIN 3 G | FAT 12 G | SATURATED FAT 6 G
SODIUM 35 MG | POTASSIUM 160 MG | FIBER 4 G | CALCIUM 25 MG
PHOSPHORUS 58 MG | IRON 1 MG

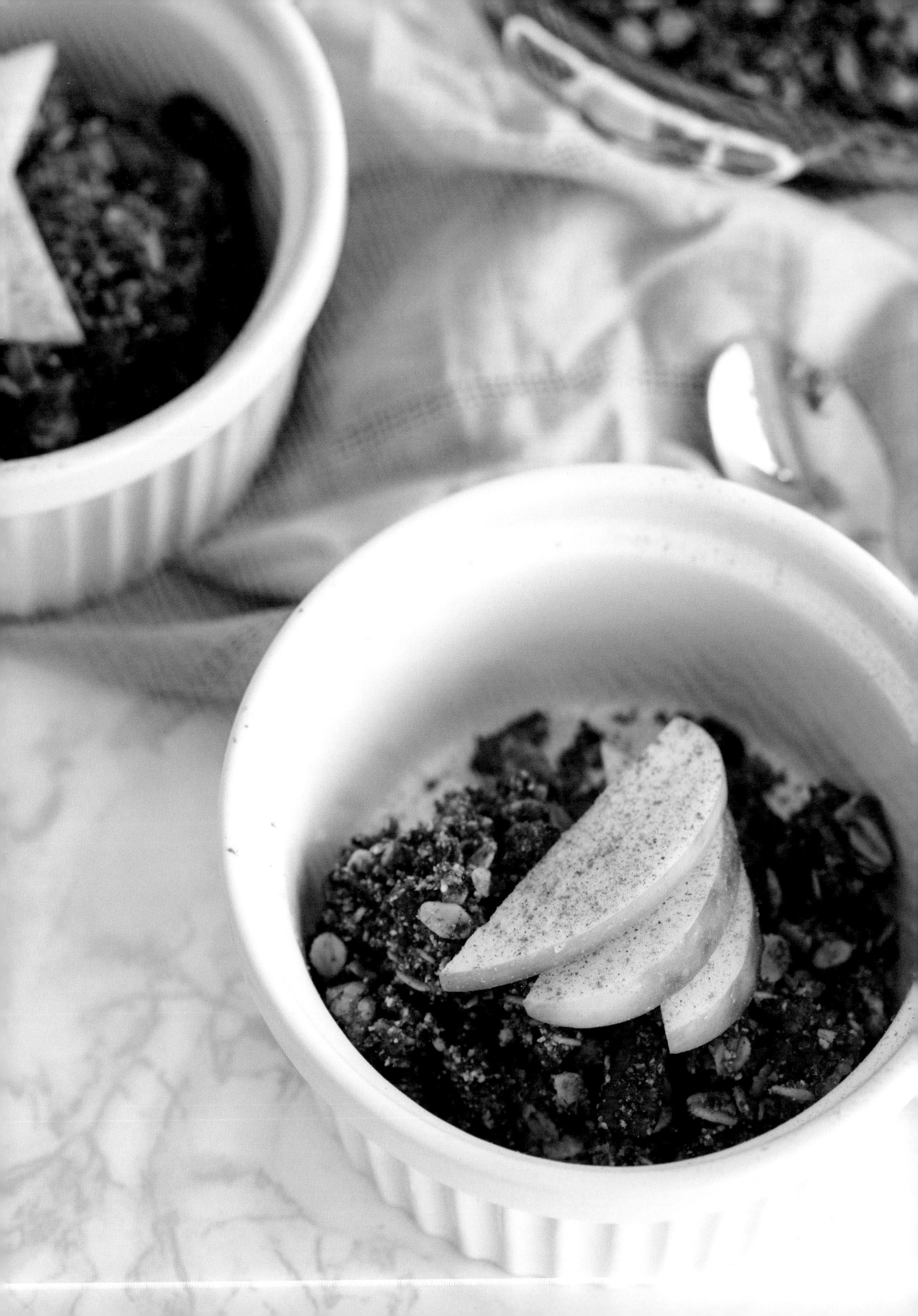

Chocolate–Avocado Pudding

DAIRY-FREE | GLUTEN-FREE | VEGAN | VEGETARIAN

YIELDS 6 SERVINGS

Ingredients

2 ripe avocados, pits removed
¼ cup cacao powder
½ cup almond milk
¼ cup pure maple syrup
½ tsp salt

Toppings

1 Tbsp coconut flakes
1 Tbsp cacao nibs
1 Tbsp hemp seeds
1 Tbsp goji berries or pumpkin seeds

Directions

1. Blend all filling ingredients on high until creamy and smooth.
2. Serve in bowls or cups of your choice and top with your preferred toppings.
3. Store in the refrigerator for up to 5 days.

KCALS 182 | CARBOHYDRATE 18 G | PROTEIN 4 G | FAT 13 G | SATURATED FAT 3 G
SODIUM 228 MG | POTASSIUM 414 MG | FIBER 6 G | CALCIUM 56 MG
PHOSPHORUS 91 MG | IRON 3 MG

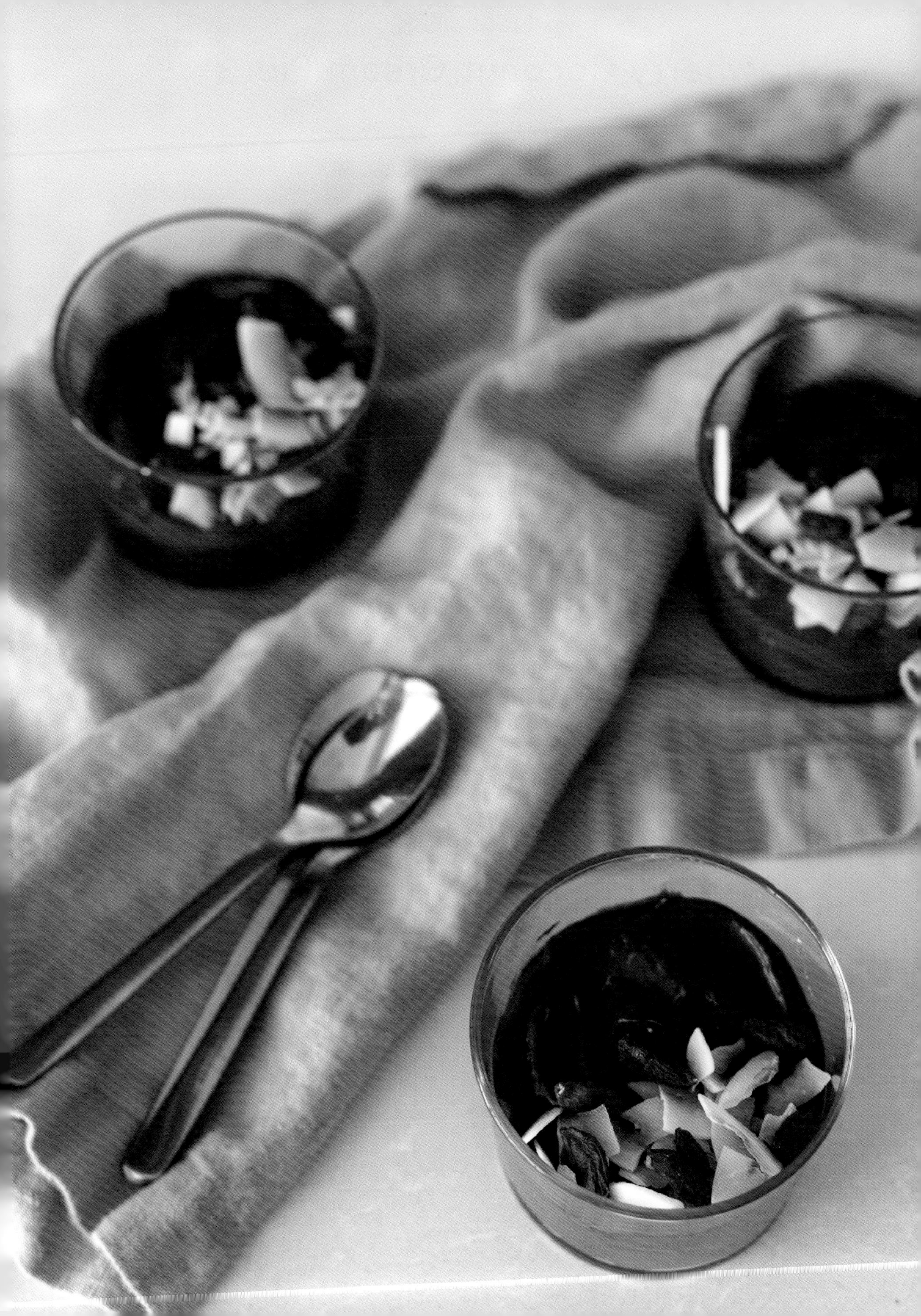

Strawberry Coconut Cream Pie

DAIRY-FREE | GLUTEN-FREE | VEGAN | VEGETARIAN

YIELDS 16 SERVINGS

Crust Ingredients

3 cups of cashew flour
¼ cup pure maple syrup, honey, or agave
3 Tbsp melted coconut oil

Filling & Topping Ingredients

2 14-oz cans coconut cream, refrigerated overnight
1/3 cup pure maple syrup, honey, or agave
1 tsp pure vanilla extract
1 lb fresh strawberries, sliced

Optional Toppings

Toasted coconut flakes
Grated dark chocolate

Directions

1. If you are making your own cashew flour, you will need to blend about ½ cup of cashews at a time. If you blend more than ½ cup at a time, it will turn into cashew butter instead of flour. So, blend ½ cup on high until all of the cashews are ground into powder, which is a matter of seconds. Dump it into a bowl and then add another ½ cup, until you reach a total of 3 cups. (If you prefer to not make your own cashew flour, you can buy almond meal at the store and use that instead; it just won't be exactly the same.)
2. Once you have your cashew flour in a mixing bowl, add all of the remaining crust ingredients into the bowl and combine until you have a thick cookie-like dough. You will probably have to use your hands to make it stick together.
3. Using a tart or cheesecake pan, firmly press the crust down into the pan, making it as even as possible. Then set it in the freezer to set.
4. Prepare the filling: Remove coconut cream from the fridge. Scoop out the solid white part and place it in the bowl of a stand mixer (a hand mixer would work, too!). Add maple syrup and vanilla, and whip until combined, smooth, and fluffy, about 1–2 minutes. It should form stiff peaks.

Directions continued →

KCALS 359 | CARBOHYDRATE 18 G | PROTEIN 7 G | FAT 32 G | SATURATED FAT 20 G
SODIUM 6 MG | POTASSIUM 394 MG | FIBER 4 G | CALCIUM 74 MG
PHOSPHORUS 171 MG | IRON 2 MG

5. Assemble: Remove crust from the freezer. Pour the filling on top, smoothing out the top with a spatula. Set in the freezer for 10 minutes.
6. Remove from freezer and top with strawberries and other desired toppings. Place back in the freezer for up to 1 hour.
7. Remove from freezer and carefully remove the pie from the pan. Place on a plate or cutting board so you can cut and serve. Store covered in the fridge for up to 7 days.

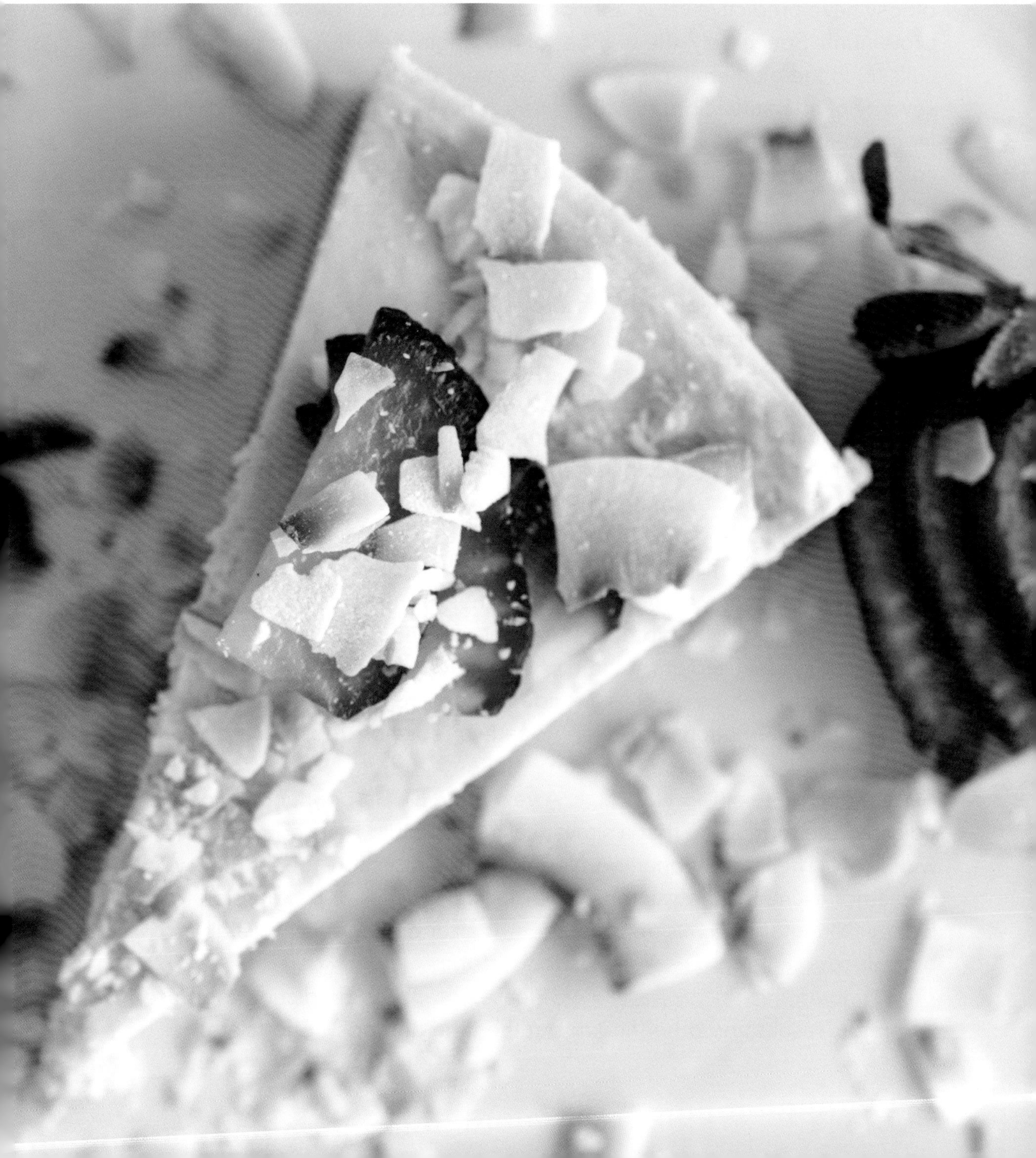

APPENDIX A

As mentioned in Dr. Julian's earlier discussion, in 2009 an international group of nephrologists and pathologists discovered that the findings of a kidney biopsy have predictive value, independent of clinical information such as proteinuria. Specifically, the number of mesangial cells (M) and endocapillary cells (E) in the glomeruli, presence of segmental sclerosis in a glomerulus, severity of interstitial fibrosis / tubular atrophy (T), and presence of glomerular crescents (C) are each important for predicting long-term kidney outcomes. These findings make up the MEST-C Oxford Classification: M score (normal = M0 vs. increased = M1), E score (normal = E0 vs. increased = E1), S score (absent = S0 vs. present = S1), T score (normal = T0 vs. moderate = T1 vs. severe = T2), and C score (absent/normal = C0 vs. mild/moderate = C1 vs. severe = C2) (Figure 5). A score above zero for each feature indicates an independent increased risk for loss of kidney function.

In 2019 Dr. Sean Barbour and colleagues combined the MEST-C scores with standard clinical information at the time of kidney biopsy of persons age 18 years and older to develop the International IgA Nephropathy Prediction Tool. This calculation estimates the risk of a 50% loss of eGFR or development of kidney failure for selected intervals up to 80 months after the kidney biopsy. The clinical information includes eGFR, systolic and diastolic blood pressures, proteinuria, age, race, and whether an angiotensin converting-enzyme inhibitor (ACEi), angiotensin receptor blocker (ARB) or an immunosuppressive drug was used at the time of or before the kidney biopsy. The estimate of the risk can be used as a guide for consideration of treatment options. The International IgA Nephropathy Prediction Tool is available at https://qxmd.com/calculate/calculator_839/international-igan-prediction-tool-post-biopsy-adults. A year later, Dr. Barbour and colleagues adjusted the formula so that a similar calculator could be used for children with IgAN. The International IgA Nephropathy Prediction Tool at Biopsy-Pediatrics estimates the risk for a 30% decline in eGFR or progression to kidney failure for intervals up to 80 months after biopsy. It is available at https://qxmd.com/calculate/calculator_713/international-igan-prediction-tool-at-biopsy-pediatrics. Please note, both prediction tools use laboratory results and other findings at the time of biopsy. Efforts are underway to further tweak the formulas in these prediction tools so that prognosis at one or two years after kidney biopsy can be estimated. By a couple of years after biopsy, many IgAN patients will have started treatment to reduce proteinuria that should slow the loss of kidney function. At the time of publication of this cookbook, we were awaiting dissemination of both updated prediction tools.

Panels A-E

Examples of kidney biopsy findings with scores greater than zero in the MEST-C Oxford Classification.

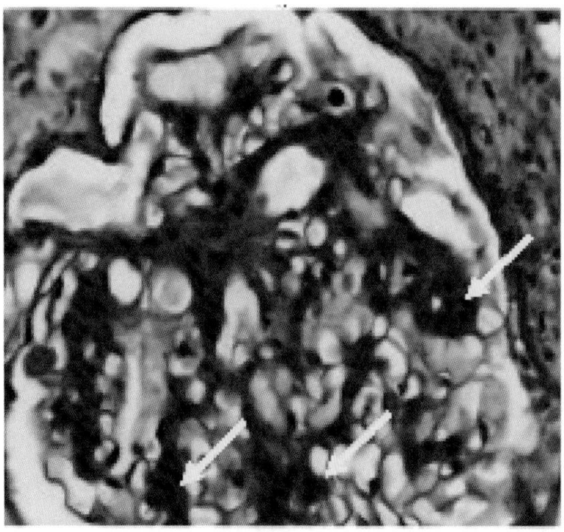

Panel A. Increased number of mesangial cells (mesangial hypercellularity) in a glomerulus. Oxford Classification, M0 = ≤ 50% glomeruli with increased number of mesangial cells, M1 = > 50% glomeruli with increased number of mesangial cells.

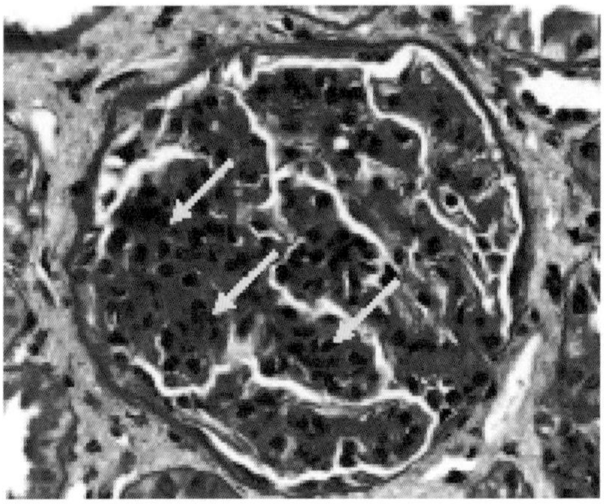

Panel B. Increased number of endocapillary cells (endocapillary hypercellularity) in a glomerulus. Oxford Classification, E0 = no glomerulus with increased number of endocapillary cells, E1 = at least one glomerulus with increased number of endocapillary cells.

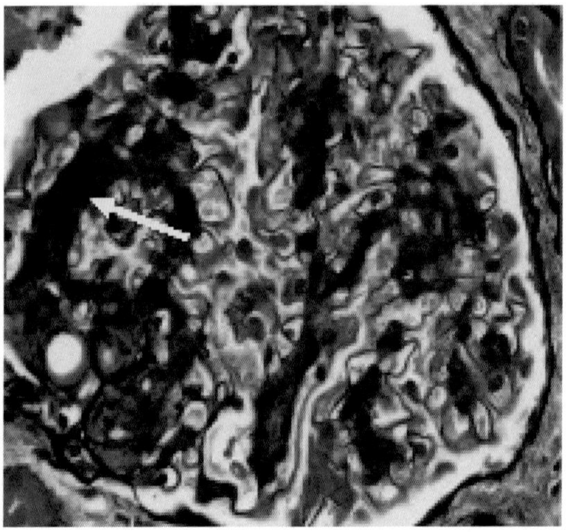

Panel C. Segmental sclerosis (scarring) in a glomerulus. Oxford Classification, S0 = no glomerulus with segmental sclerosis, S1 = at least one glomerulus with segmental sclerosis.

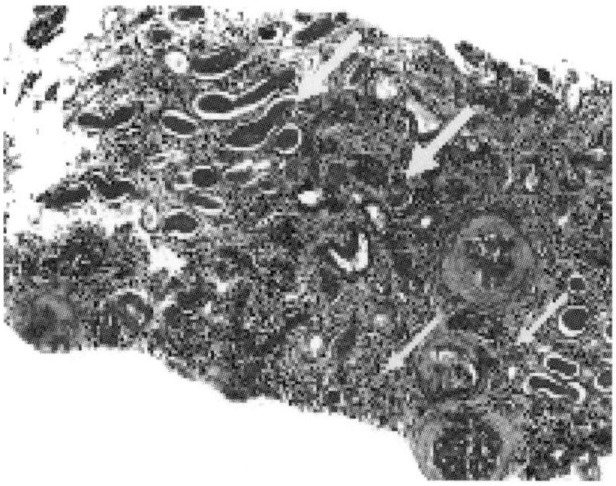

Panel D. Interstitial fibrosis (scarring) indicated by thin arrows and tubular atrophy by thick arrows. Oxford Classification, T0 = 0–25% of cortical area affected, T1 = 26–50% of cortical area affected, and T2 = > 50% cortical area affected.

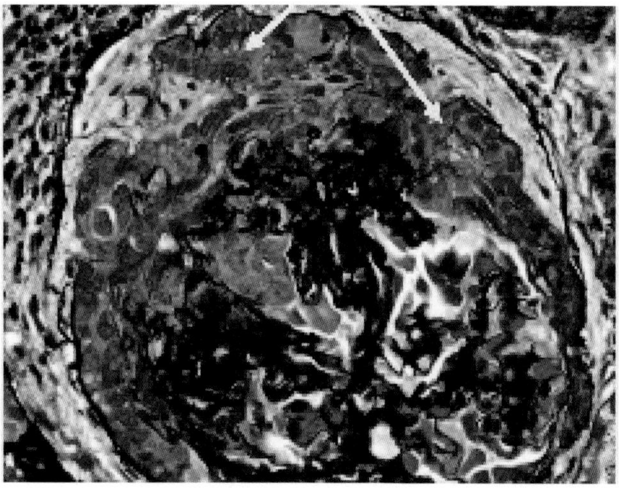

Panel E. Crescent filling much of the urinary space around the tuft of capillaries of a glomerulus. Oxford Classification, C0 = no glomerulus with crescent, C1 = crescent present in 1–24% of glomeruli, C2 = crescent in ≥ 25% of glomeruli.